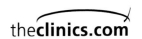

DENTAL CLINICS
OF NORTH AMERICA

Contemporary Dental and
Maxillofacial Imaging

GUEST EDITORS
Steven L. Thomas, DDS, MS
Christos Angelopoulos, DDS, MS

October 2008 • Volume 52 • Number 4

SAUNDERS

An Imprint of Elsevier, Inc.
PHILADELPHIA LONDON TORONTO MONTREAL SYDNEY TOKYO

W.B. SAUNDERS COMPANY
A Division of Elsevier Inc.

1600 John F. Kennedy Boulevard • Suite 1800 • Philadelphia, Pennsylvania 19103-2899

http://www.dental.theclinics.com

DENTAL CLINICS OF NORTH AMERICA
October 2008
Editor: John Vassallo; j.vassallo@elsevier.com

Volume 52, Number 4
ISSN 0011-8532
ISBN-13: 978-1-4160-6286-8
ISBN-10: 1-4160-6286-6

Photocopying

Single photocopies of single articles may be made for personal use as allowed by national copyright laws. Permission of the Publisher and payment of a fee is required for all other photocopying, including multiple or systematic copying, copying for advertising or promotional purposes, resale, and all forms of document delivery. Special rates are available for educational institutions that wish to make photocopies for non-profit educational classroom use. For information on how to seek permission visit www.elsevier.com/permissions or call: (+44) 1865 843830 (UK)/(+1) 215 239 3804 (USA).

Derivative Works

Subscribers may reproduce tables of contents or prepare lists of articles including abstracts for internal circulation within their institutions. Permission of the Publisher is required for resale or distribution outside the institution. Permission of the Publisher is required for all other derivative works, including compilations and translations (please consult www.elsevier.com/permissions).

Electronic Storage or Usage

Permission of the Publisher is required to store or use electronically any material contained in this journal, including any article or part of an article (please consult www.elsevier.com/permissions). Except as outlined above, no part of this publication may be reproduced, stored in a retrieval system or transmitted in any form or by any means, electronic, mechanical, photocopying, recording or otherwise, without prior written permission of the Publisher.

Notice

No responsibility is assumed by the Publisher for any injury and/or damage to persons or property as a matter of products liability, negligence or otherwise, or from any use or operation of any methods, products, instructions or ideas contained in the material herein. Because of rapid advances in the medical sciences, in particular, independent verification of diagnoses and drug dosages should be made.

Although all advertising material is expected to conform to ethical (medical) standards, inclusion in this publication does not constitute a guarantee or endorsement of the quality or value of such product or of the claims made of it by its manufacturer.

Dental Clinics of North America (ISSN 0011-8532) is published quarterly by Elsevier Inc., 360 Park Avenue South, New York, NY 10010-1710. Months of issue are January, April, July, and October. Business and Editorial Offices: 1600 John F. Kennedy Boulevard, Suite 1800, Philadelphia, PA 19103-2899. Customer Service Office: 6277 Sea Harbor Drive, Orlando, FL 32887-4800. Periodicals postage paid at New York, NY and additional mailing offices. Subscription prices are $207.00 per year (domestic individual), $347.00 per year (domestic institution), $100.00 per year (domestic student/resident), $246.00 per year (Canadian individual), $437.00 per year (Canadian institution), $297.00 per year (international individual), $437.00 per year (international institution), and $150.00 per year (international and Canadian student/resident, $99.00 (single issue non-subscriber). International air speed delivery is included in all *Clinics* subscription prices. All prices are subject to change without notice. **POSTMASTER:** Send address changes to *Dental Clinics of North America*, Elsevier Periodicals Customer Service, 6277 Sea Harbor Drive, Orlando, FL 32887-4800. Customer Service: 1-800-654-2452 (US). From outside the United States, call 1-407-563-6020. Fax: 1-407-363-9661. E-mail: JournalsCustomerService-usa@elsevier.com.

Reprints: For copies of 100 or more of articles in this publication, please contact the Commercial Reprints Department, Elsevier Inc., 360 Park Avenue South, New York, NY 10010-1710. Tel.: 212-633-3812; Fax: 212-462-1935; E-mail: reprints@elsevier.com.

The *Dental Clinics of North America* is covered in *MEDLINE/PubMed (Index Medicus)*, *Current Contents/Clinical Medicine*, *ISI/BIOMED* and *Clinahl*.

Printed in the United States of America.

GUEST EDITORS

STEVEN L. THOMAS, DDS, MS, MD*, Thomas Oral Surgery, PC, Overland Park, Kansas

CHRISTOS ANGELOPOULOS, DDS, MS, Associate Professor and Director, Division of Oral and Maxillofacial Radiology, Columbia University, College of Dental Medicine, New York, New York

CONTRIBUTORS

SHELLY ABRAMOWICZ, DMD, Resident, Department of Oral and Maxillofacial Surgery, University of Florida College of Dentistry, Gainesville, Florida

CHRISTOS ANGELOPOULOS, DDS, MS, Associate Professor and Director, Division of Oral and Maxillofacial Radiology, Columbia University, College of Dental Medicine, New York, New York

COREY C. BURGOYNE, DMD, Chief Resident, Department of Oral and Maxillofacial Surgery, Virginia Commonwealth University Medical Center, Medical College of Virginia Hospitals, Richmond, Virginia

M. FRANKLIN DOLWICK, DMD, PhD, Professor and Chairman, Department of Oral and Maxillofacial Surgery, University of Florida College of Dentistry, Gainesville, Florida

ALLAN G. FARMAN, BDS, PhD, DSc, MBA, Professor and Director, Radiology and Imaging Sciences, Department of Surgical/Hospital Dentistry, University of Louisville School of Dentistry, Louisville, Kentucky

SCOTT D. GANZ, DMD, Prosthodontics, Maxillofacial Prosthetics & Implant Dentistry, Fort Lee; Clinical Assistant Professor, Department of Restorative Dentistry, University of Medicine and Dentistry of New Jersey, Newark, New Jersey

STEVEN A. GUTTENBERG, DDS, MD, Director, Washington Institute for Mouth, Face and Jaw Surgery; Senior Attending Surgeon and Chairman of the Training and Education Committee, Department of Oral and Maxillofacial Surgery, Washington Hospital Center, Washington, District of Columbia; Professor of Surgery, Nova Southeastern University College of Dental Medicine, Fort Lauderdale, Florida; Professor of Surgery, Temple University, Philadelphia, Pennsylvania

STEVEN L. HECHLER, DDS, MS, Overland Park, Kansas

EMMA L. LEWIS, BDS, MBBS, Assistant Professor, Department of Oral and Maxillofacial Surgery, University of Florida College of Dentistry, Gainesville, Florida

DALE A. MILES, DDS, MS, FRCD(C), Adjunct Professor, University of Texas at San Antonio, San Antonio, Texas; Arizona School of Dentistry and Oral Health, Mesa, Arizona

MICHAEL J. PHAROAH, DDS, MSc, FRCD(C), Professor, Department of Radiology, Faculty of Dentistry, University of Toronto, Toronto, Ontario, Canada

SONALI RATHORE, BDS, Graduate Student, Division of Oral and Maxillofacial Radiology, University of North Carolina School of Dentistry, Chapel Hill, North Carolina

STEPHANIE L. REEDER, DMD, Resident, Department of Oral and Maxillofacial Surgery, University of Florida College of Dentistry, Gainesville, Florida

WILLIAM C. SCARFE, BDS, FRACDS, MS, Professor, Radiology and Imaging Sciences, Department of Surgical/Hospital Dentistry, University of Louisville School of Dentistry, Louisville, Kentucky

LEONARD SPECTOR, DDS, Spector + Krupp, DDS, PA, Oral and Maxillofacial Surgery, Towson, Maryland

ROBERT A. STRAUSS, DDS, MD, Professor, and Director of Residency Training Program, Department of Oral and Maxillofacial Surgery, Virginia Commonwealth University Medical Center, Medical College of Virginia Hospitals, Richmond, Virginia

STEVEN L. THOMAS, DDS, MS, MD*, Thomas Oral Surgery, PC, Overland Park, Kansas

DONALD A. TYNDALL, DDS, MSPH, PhD, Professor of Diagnostic Sciences and General Dentistry, and Director, Division of Oral and Maxillofacial Radiology, University of North Carolina School of Dentistry, Chapel Hill, North Carolina

STUART C. WHITE, DDS, PhD, Professor, Section of Oral and Maxillofacial Radiology, University of California, Los Angeles School of Dentistry, Los Angeles, California

* *Not licensed to practice medicine*

CONTENTS

During the last decades, an exciting new array of imaging modalities, such as digital imaging, CT, MRI, positron emission tomography, and cone-beam CT (CBCT), has provided astounding new images that continually contribute to the accuracy of diagnostic tasks of the maxillofacial region. The most recent, cone-beam imaging, is gaining rapid acceptance in dentistry because it provides cross-sectional imaging that is often a valuable supplement to intraoral and panoramic radiographs. The information content in such examinations is high and the dose and costs are low. The increasing trend toward the use of CBCT in dental offices may be expected to result in improved diagnosis, but with increased patient dose and health care costs. Using CBCT as a secondary imaging tool helps optimize health-to-risk ratio.

This article on x-ray cone-beam CT (CBCT) acquisition provides an overview of the fundamental principles of operation of this technology and the influence of geometric and software parameters on image quality and patient radiation dose. Advantages of the CBCT system and a summary of the uses and limitations of the images produced are discussed. All current generations of CBCT systems provide useful diagnostic images. Future enhancements most likely will be directed toward reducing scan time; providing multimodal imaging; improving image fidelity, including soft tissue contrast; and incorporating task-specific protocols to minimize patient dose.

FORTHCOMING ISSUES

RECENT ISSUES

THE DENTAL
CLINICS
OF NORTH AMERICA

Dent Clin N Am 52 (2008) xi–xii

Preface

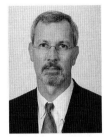 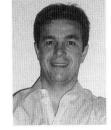

Steven L. Thomas, DDS, MS   Christos Angelopoulos, DDS, MS
Guest Editors

Although nothing can replace history and physical examination when evaluating patients, the use and evolution of non-invasive technology for imaging areas not visible to the human eye has become a bigger part of the diagnostic process. Dental imaging has advanced rapidly over the last years. Static projectional images were relied upon for diagnoses in the maxillofacial region, but we are moving toward digital, three-dimensional (3D) and interactive imaging applications. Much of this movement is attributed to a recently introduced CT technology known as "cone-beam computed tomography" or "digital volume tomography." This technology has offered dentists a view of all angles of areas of concern. This technology has been embraced quickly by the dental profession. It is considered as "what was missing" by many in the field.

3D imaging has improved diagnostic efficiency and the practice of dentistry in a variety of ways; from routine evaluation to complex analysis of unusual pathology and congenital deformities, the technology available today makes dentistry better, and easier, and more accurate. At the same time, a plethora of applications have been developed that use the three-dimensional data for a variety of tasks: implant planning, surgical navigation, orthodontic applications, and more. All of this is for the benefit of patients.

Dental Clinics of North America always is committed to presenting advances in the dental field and has honored us with the charge to assemble a panel of experts to present a broad view of the advancements in maxillofacial imaging and the various applications of 3D imaging in dentistry. We

doi:10.1016/j.cden.2008.07.003   *dental.theclinics.com*

thank the *Dental Clinics of North America* for this honor. We also thank all of the authors who contributed to this issue; all of them are recognized experts in their field.

Lastly, several brand names of software applications and solutions are mentioned throughout this issue. The use of such software programs reflects the personal preference of the author(s) and is neither a recommendation nor an endorsement by the guest editors and the publisher. We recommend a thorough search for evidence before deciding to incorporate one or more of these applications in one's practice.

We sincerely hope you will be stimulated and challenged by what you read in this issue and that you will find the information useful in caring for your patients.

Steven L. Thomas, DDS, MS
Thomas Oral Surgery, PC
12800 Metcalf Avenue, Suite 2
Overland Park, KS 66213, USA

E-mail address: thomas@thomasoralsurgery.com

Christos Angelopoulos, DDS, MS
Division of Oral and Maxillofacial Radiology
Columbia University
College of Dental Medicine
PH-7 Stem-134
New York, NY 10032, USA

E-mail address: ca2291@columbia.edu

ELSEVIER
SAUNDERS

THE DENTAL
CLINICS
OF NORTH AMERICA

Dent Clin N Am 52 (2008) 689–705

The Evolution and Application of Dental Maxillofacial Imaging Modalities

Stuart C. White, DDS, PhD[a],*,
Michael J. Pharoah, DDS, MSc, FRCD(C)[b]

[a]*Section of Oral and Maxillofacial Radiology, University of California, Los Angeles School of Dentistry, 10833 Le Conte Avenue, Los Angeles, CA 90095-1668, USA*
[b]*Department of Radiology, Faculty of Dentistry, University of Toronto, 124 Edward Street, Toronto, Ontario M5G 1G6, Canada*

Dental radiology has long played an exciting and critical diagnostic role in dentistry, never truer than now with the rapidly expanding array of imaging modalities. Intraoral radiography was first used within weeks of the discovery of X rays by Roentgen in 1895. Extraoral imaging, including cephalometric radiography, followed soon thereafter. Panoramic radiography has provided broad coverage of the teeth and surrounding structures since the mid-twentieth century. Each of these modalities has adapted to the digital revolution. Recent decades have seen the development of CT, MRI, nuclear medicine, and ultrasonography, imaging modalities that have revolutionized dental and medical diagnosis. CT can be simply defined as the use of the X ray–based imaging method to produce three-dimensional (3D) images usually displayed in the form of image slices. The original CT technology, which is used extensively in medical diagnosis, is designated as medical CT (CT) and the newer modality used primarily in dentistry is cone-beam CT (CBCT). The recent development and application of cone-beam imaging in dentistry provides most of the benefits of CT imaging for many dental applications at a substantial savings of dose and cost. This introductory article provides an overview of the imaging principles underlying each of these technologies, identifies dental applications, and, in particular, focuses on the emerging role of cone-beam imaging in dentistry. Some areas of CBCT that need further attention are also considered. Conventional tomography has been substantially replaced by CBCT and is not considered.

* Corresponding author.
  E-mail address: swhite@ucla.edu (S.C. White).

0011-8532/08/$ - see front matter © 2008 Elsevier Inc. All rights reserved.
doi:10.1016/j.cden.2008.05.006 *dental.theclinics.com*

Periapical radiography

Conventional intraoral periapical and bitewing radiographs are familiar and ubiquitous, and, when well made, they provide excellent images for most dental radiographic needs. Their primary use is to supplement the clinical examination by providing insight into the internal structure of teeth and supporting bone to reveal caries, alveolar bone loss associated with periodontal disease, periapical disease, and a wide range of other dental and osseous conditions.

Intraoral imaging

Intraoral imaging still provides the best spatial resolution of any imaging method. However, as a result of collapsing 3D structural information onto a two-dimensional (2D) image, spatial information is lost in the third dimension. For instance, does the radiolucency seen on the crown of a lower first molar come from a lesion in the buccal pit or on the occlusal surface? What is the relationship of the unerupted mandibular third molar to the mandibular canal? The clinician must attempt to reconstruct mentally this 2D image into a 3D reality with limited information from 2D images.

Film

Film is highly flexible, literally and figuratively. Well-processed film radiographs offer highly detailed images at a low cost. Unfortunately, film processing is often suboptimal, with deleterious consequences to image quality. Furthermore, maintaining a darkroom requires space and time and has environmental costs.

Digital

During the last decade, many dental practices replaced film with digital imaging systems. Common reasons for making this transition included improved patient education, lower exposure, greater speed of obtaining images, and the perception of being up to date in the eyes of patients [1]. Two broad types of digital systems are commercially available for dental offices. Most common are the solid-state sensors, made using either charge-coupled device (CCD) or complementary metal oxide semiconductor (CMOS) technology. The alternative technology is photostimulable phosphor (PSP) plates, also called storage phosphor plates.

Charge-coupled device–complementary metal oxide semiconductor

These systems use rigid sensors placed intraorally to capture the image. A cable usually connects the sensor to the computer. When a radiograph is made, the remnant x-ray beam exiting the patient is captured in a scintillator coating a silicon chip. The scintillator immediately re-emits visible light photons that cause electrons to be released within the silicon chip, resulting in a voltage differential. The amount of the voltage is proportional to the exposure. The smallest unit from which a voltage can be recorded corresponds to a pixel, the smallest picture element. Although the actual voltages in a series of pixels may comprise a continuous spectrum, an analog signal, they are converted to a more limited set of 256, 1024, or more specific (digital) values. This image information is optimized by proprietary software and the resulting image is displayed on a computer monitor within seconds of the exposure.

Photostimulable phosphor

PSP systems use imaging plates to capture an image. These plates are typically thinner than solid-state sensors, have no wires, and are flexible. When an image is made using a PSP system, x-ray photons strike a phosphor coating on the plate and cause electrons to be stored in a higher energy state. Following the exposure, the plate is removed from the patient's mouth and placed in a laser reader for scanning. When a laser light is directed onto the exposed plate, the electrons return to their ground state and release visible light. This amount of light, which is proportional to the exposure, is read in a photomultiplier tube. The analog signal is digitized, optimized, and displayed on a monitor, as with the solid-state detectors. This process takes from a few seconds to a few minutes.

Clinical considerations

Because film, the CCD-CMOS, and PSP systems all offer essentially equivalent diagnostic information, a decision to "go digital" is made for other reasons. One of the more important reasons for using digital imaging is to facilitate patient education. Displaying a large image on a computer screen provides dentists an excellent opportunity to educate patients regarding their condition and treatment needs. Other important benefits of digital imaging include a reduced chance of losing films and the fact that images can be transferred easily by e-mail, especially useful for second opinions.

The CCD-CMOS systems provide almost immediate images with the sensor still in the mouth, which allows the operator to examine the resulting image, make any adjustments in orientation of the sensor or x-ray aiming tube that may be required for a retake, or proceed to the next exposure, often without having to remove the sensor from the mouth. This consideration is an important one for endodontists. In contrast, with the PSP systems, the sensor must be removed from the mouth after each exposure, as with film. This system is thus more analogous to film and is fully appropriate for restorative dentistry. It is best to scan the plates soon after exposure because the latent image decays with time.

The rigidity of the CCD-CMOS sensors may cause difficulties in positioning the sensor in the patient's mouth, in terms of patient discomfort and displaying the desired anatomy. This problem is particularly acute in offices where the patient traditionally holds a flexible film in his/her mouth while an exposure is made. The best means to position the sensor is to use holders that can support the sensor deep in the patient's mouth, well away from the teeth being imaged. This technique will allow the apical end of the sensor to capture tooth apices and surrounding bone with minimal discomfort to the patient. Furthermore, the sensor holder should have an external guide to allow accurate positioning of the x-ray tube head. On the other hand, the flexibility of some of the PSP plates may lead to image distortion if the patient bends it while holding it in the mouth with his/her finger. Again, it is best to use a holder that supports the plate in the middle of the mouth parallel to the teeth, and which has an external guide ring for aligning the x-ray head.

The choice of a digital system can be influenced by costs. CCD and CMOS systems require an initial cash outlay for sensors of several thousands of dollars each. A PSP laser reader costs approximately $10,000 and the plates cost a few tens of dollars each. Both systems may have additional costs for software and computer equipment. Unlike film, PSP plates can be reused, although they may become scratched and require replacement.

Image processing

An often-touted advantage of digital systems is the ability to use image-processing tools such as brightness, contrast, and sharpening routines to improve image interpretation. Although such tools may indeed improve the subjective appearance of images, evidence is scant of improved disease detection or diagnosis given a well-exposed initial image. Indeed, if these tools are applied improperly, degradation of an image, potentially leading to inaccurate interpretation, is a real possibility.

Dose

Many exaggerated advertising claims have been made about dose reduction with digital imaging. The consensus is that CCD and CMOS systems do require somewhat less exposure than F-speed film. However, difficulties with use typically prompt more images to be made than when film is used, thus obviating their dose advantage. PSP plates present another interesting situation. These plates have broad image latitude and are thus able to accept unnecessarily high radiation exposures and still display high-quality images. Care must be taken to assure that low exposures, essentially the same as those used for F-speed film, are used, to avoid unnecessary overexposure of the patient.

Data management

With all digital systems, it is critical to plan for adequate data storage and backup capabilities for the patient management and digital imaging systems. It is often useful to send images to an insurance carrier or a colleague. To accomplish this, images can typically be exported into a nonproprietary format such as JPEG or TIF and sent as e-mail attachments. Images can also be printed onto thermal film or papers but they often lose image quality in this process.

Panoramic imaging

Panoramic imaging has been evolving continuously since its introduction in the 1950s. The basic imaging principle is that of curved surface tomography. A narrow, vertical x-ray beam is directed through the patient's head. The exit beam then passes through a slit in a shield on the opposite side, where it is captured on a receptor, either film or digital. The x-ray source and film rotate synchronously around the patient's head. The receptor also travels behind the shield as it rotates around the patient. The image shows on the receptor side of the patient because the rate and direction that the receptor travels behind the shield is the same as the rate at which the x-ray beam passes through the teeth and other structures on the receptor side of the patient. This process results in a sharp image of the teeth and bone on the film side of the patient, whereas structures on the tube side are blurred beyond recognition. The patient doses from CCD and PSP systems are comparable to those received from film/intensifying screens. The resolution of all systems is comparable.

Film

Film has been used in panoramic machines since its inception and always in combination with matching intensifying screens. These screens contain rare-earth elements and fluoresce green or blue light when struck by x-ray photons. This light exposes the silver bromide crystals in the film and forms the latent image that is subsequently made visible by film processing.

Charge-coupled device

CCD sensors have been used in recent years to capture the image in some panoramic machines. A 6 in × 12 in sensor is too expensive to manufacture; a linear array, approximately 4 pixels wide, is used to capture the image. This linear CCD array is read out continuously as the exposure is being made, thus building up the image from one side to the other. The image data are then stored on a hard disk and may be displayed on a monitor.

Storage phosphor plates

PSP technology is also used to acquire panoramic images. In this case, large plates, approximately 6 in × 12 in, are used. The plates are exposed and then read in a laser reader. The resultant image is displayed on a computer monitor and stored like other images.

Clinical considerations

Panoramic radiography is excellent in providing an overview of oral hard tissues, including presence and location of teeth, foreign bodies, cysts, tumors, and other conditions within the jaws. The resolution of panoramic images is sufficient for many dental tasks but less than that provided by intraoral imaging and thus may be insufficient to reveal early or subtle disease. Panoramic radiographs are most useful when full coverage of the jaws is desired or when a specific region that is too large to be seen on a periapical view is desired. For many patients not having extensive dental disease, a thorough clinical examination accompanied by a panoramic view plus four bitewings serves as a good initial examination. Then, on the basis of these images and clinical findings, additional supplemental periapical views may be indicated [2].

The major advantages of panoramic images are the broad coverage of oral structures, the low patient dose (about 10% of a full-mouth examination), and the moderately low cost of the equipment (compared with cone-beam imaging [see later discussion]). Some newer panoramic machines incorporate cone-beam technology.

The major limitations of panoramic imaging are the reduced resolution compared with intraoral images and the fact that the focal trough is fairly thick, enough to see the full thickness of the alveolar ridges, and thus it presents essentially a 2D projection image of these regions. Also, image distortion and the presence of phantom images of anatomy outside the focal trough, such as overlapping cervical spine images on the anterior maxilla and mandible, can artificially produce apparent changes or may hide significant findings.

Cone-beam imaging

CBCT has gained broad acceptance in dentistry in the last 5 years, although its roots go back about 2 decades. The major innovation compared with intraoral and panoramic imaging is that it provides high-quality, thin-slice images. Cone-beam machines emit an x-ray beam shaped liked a cone, rather than a fan, as in conventional CT machines. Because the beam covers the entire region of interest, it is only necessary for the x-ray source to make one pass or less around the patient's head, when acquiring images. The beam exiting the patient is captured on a 2D planar detector, usually an amorphous silicon flat panel or sometimes an image intensifier/CCD detector. The beam diameter ranges from 4 cm to 30 cm. As the x-ray source goes around the patient's head, the sensor captures from 160 to 599 basis images. These images are used to compute a spherical or cylindric volume including all, or a portion of, the face. In this volume, the densities at all locations (voxels) are calculated from the basis images. Voxels are cuboids and can be as small as 0.125 mm. Typically, serial cross-sectional views are made in the axial, sagittal, and coronal planes (Fig. 1). From this data set, the operator can also extract thick or thin, planar or curved reconstructions in any orientation. Furthermore, true 3D images of bone or soft tissue surfaces can be generated. This article considers clinical uses of large and small field-of-view machines and emerging usage issues. Other articles in this issue provide more detailed information regarding this technology and its applications.

Special-purpose, third-party software is being developed continuously that uses the data generated by cone-beam units and typically provides display and measuring tools for specific purposes. These programs may be sophisticated and their capabilities may far exceed those of the software supplied with the CBCT machine. When a dentist wants to use such software, the processed volumetric data are exported from the CBCT manufacturer's software as a Digital Imaging and Communications in Medicine (DICOM) data set. These data may then be imported into the third-party software for

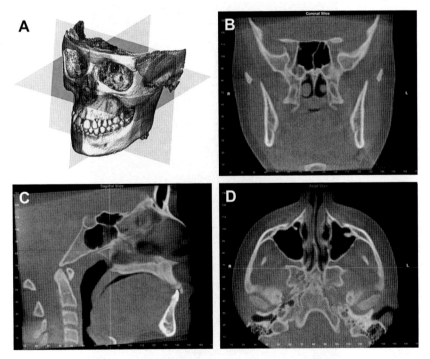

Fig. 1. Standard display modes of CBCT volumetric data. (*A*) Volumetric 3D hard tissue showing the three orthogonal planes in relation to the reconstructed volumetric data set: coronal, sagittal, and axial. Each orthogonal plane has multiple thin-slice sections in each plane. (*B*) Representative coronal image, (*C*) representative sagittal image, and (*D*) representative axial image. Images produced using Dolphin 3D, Chatsworth, California. (*From* White SC, Pharoah MJ. Oral radiology, principles and interpretation. 6th edition. St. Louis (MO): Mosby; in press; with permission.)

analysis. Most such software has been developed for assisting in implants treatment planning and for orthodontics, for display of relationships between hard and soft tissues (Fig. 2) and for making measurements of true distances and angles. The data set generated by cone-beam imaging can also be used to produce rapid-prototyping models for treatment planning, such as in orthognathic surgery cases, for forensic uses such as legal cases, or to build surgical guides for implant placement.

Clinical considerations

The most common indications for cone-beam imaging in dentistry are assessment of the jaws for placement of dental implants, examination of teeth and facial structures for orthodontic treatment planning, evaluation of the temporomandibular joints (TMJs) for osseous degenerative changes,

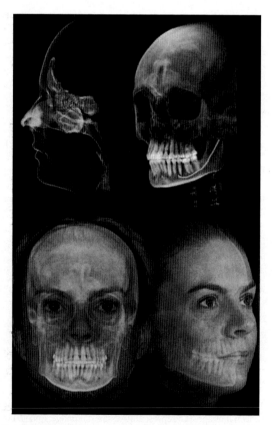

Fig. 2. Fusion. Three-dimensional anatomic views demonstrating imaging possibilities with fusion of CBCT data and photographic image sets. Images created using 3DMD, Atlanta, Georgia. (*Courtesy of* Chester Wang, Chatsworth, CA.)

evaluation of the proximity of the lower wisdom teeth to the mandibular nerve before extraction, assessment of teeth for root fracture or periapical disease, and evaluation of bone for signs of infections, cysts, or tumors. Cone-beam imaging is rapidly replacing conventional tomography for these tasks. All these applications, and many others, benefit from viewing thin slices through the region of interest without superposition of local complex anatomy onto the image.

Cone-beam machines may be broadly classified as providing large or limited imaging volumes. The large-volume machines have image fields with diameters of 6 in to up to 12 in. The limited-volume machines generate images 4 cm or 6 cm in diameter but have higher spatial resolution. The large-volume machines are more appropriate for orthodontics, full-arch implants treatment planning, or orthognathic surgery. The limited-volume machines are most appropriate for examining individual teeth for fracture or periapical disease, evaluating the relationship of third molars to the mandibular canal, single-site implant, or the osseous components of the TMJs.

The principal limitation of large-volume cone-beam imaging is the moderate resolution provided by the images compared with intraoral radiographs or the limited-volume CBCT machines. In broad terms, their image quality is comparable to that of panoramic imaging, sufficient for a broad range of tasks but insufficient for high-detail tasks, such as examining for nondisplaced fractures in teeth or small root canals. Additionally, unlike conventional CT, the contrast resolution is limited to the densities of calcified structures such as bone. Although the interface between soft tissues and air is readily identified, no soft tissue window images exist, as in CT, that enable differentiation of various soft tissues. The effective dose from large-volume machines ranges widely, from 2.7 times to 25 times a conventional panoramic examination [3].

The limited-volume instruments may provide images of high clarity, although of a limited anatomic region (Fig. 3). The clarity of these images is comparable to that of periapical films, yet with all the advantages of cross-sectional imaging in all planes. The effective dose from these machines is also low, comparable to a panoramic view or a set of bitewings.

An important limitation of large- and limited-volume cone-beam imaging and conventional CT is the presence of metallic artifacts caused by metallic restorations and, to a lesser extent, root canal filling material and implants. These artifacts appear as bright or dark streaks in the image plane containing these structures and they degrade image quality. Such artifacts may also appear as dark bands around amalgam restorations simulating recurrent caries, or as dark zones or streaks around endodontic materials simulating root fractures.

Usage issues

CBCT has been used widely in dentistry for only a few years. The first units were purchased by universities, private dental radiology practices,

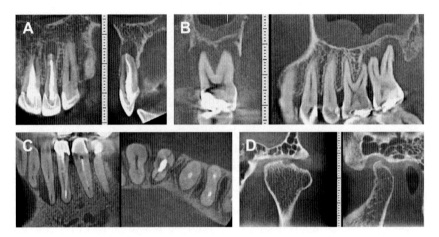

Fig. 3. Regional cone-beam imaging. Numerous dental conditions can be demonstrated in high resolution with regional CBCT, including (*A*) periapical pathology, (*B*) periodontal and periapical disease, (*C*) root fracture and associated alveolar bone loss, and (*D*) coronal and lateral views of TMJ. Images captured using 3DX Accuitomo, J. Morita Manufacturing Corp., Kyoto, Japan. (*From* White SC, Pharoah MJ. Oral radiology, principles and interpretation. 6th edition. St. Louis (MO): Mosby; in press; with permission.)

and oral radiographic laboratories. The recent trend has been for dentists, particularly those specializing in orthodontics, oral surgery, and periodontics, to purchase such machines for their practices. This trend carries potential advantages and disadvantages in terms of delivery of health care.

As cone-beam imaging becomes increasingly available in dental practice, the benefits of this imaging modality will be increasingly received. It is reasonable to anticipate that the ready availability of high-quality CBCT will improve diagnosis and treatment planning and thus lead to improved patient care and treatment outcomes. Some early studies, for instance, have described improved diagnosis of endodontic cases with limited-volume machines [4,5] and orthodontic care [6].

However, signs exist of suboptimal use of CBCT in some offices. It is possible that some practitioners will use CBCT only to make panoramic reconstructions as a substitute for conventional panoramic images. In such situations, a conventional panoramic image can been used, sparing the patient unnecessary radiation exposure. The dose to patients, individually and collectively, could be substantially reduced by using conventional panoramic images as an initial survey in such situations, and only when necessary making a well-collimated CBCT examination and cross-sectional images in the area of interest.

Many questions remain unanswered concerning the appropriate indications for CBCT examinations. In many situations, the cone-beam image provides unique and definitive information crucial to care. One challenge is to identify patients likely to benefit from cone-beam examinations and those for whom conventional imaging is adequate. Does every patient requiring orthodontic, endodontic, oral surgical, or periodontal care require a cone-beam examination? Certainly not. Similar to the introduction of other new imaging modalities such as CT and MRI, it will take clinical experience and research to determine the most effective patient application of CBCT technology. Such recommendations are already provided by the American Dental Association for conventional imaging in dentistry [7]. Although the literature of antidotal reports describing clinical applications of cone-beam imaging is expanding rapidly, few evidence-based articles have evaluated the most effective selection of patients for imaging. The clinician who has made a substantial investment to use the cone-beam examination may be tempted to use it more frequently than might be justified to help defray the expense of the machine. If such situations do occur, then the net result for the patient would be increased exposure and health care costs without increased diagnostic benefit.

Another issue that needs to be considered, particularly with the large field-of-view cone-beam images, is the training and experience of the individuals interpreting the images. Even though a particular clinician may have a specific interest, for example, placing an implant in the anterior maxilla, the CBCT field of view may extend from the middle cranial fossa and sella turcica inferiorly to the hyoid bone and as far posteriorly as the cervical spine. It is possible for various osseous or soft tissue diseases to be detected in the complex anatomy of this region. It is important to make multiplanar reconstructions through the entire volume images and to examine the entire volume image, typically in 1-mm slices in the axial, coronal, and sagittal planes. The authors of this article have detected numerous unanticipated clinically significant findings by such an examination protocol. It is our belief that, because this volume of tissue is exposed and readily available for review, the analysis must not be limited to the region of interest; rather, all the imaging information must be analyzed.

CT

CT has been useful for many years in dentistry for providing cross-sectional implant imaging for evaluating various infections, cysts, tumors, and trauma in the maxillofacial region. Unlike CBCT, in CT imaging, the x-ray source travels helically around the patient many times, emitting a narrow fan beam until the region of interest is covered [8,9]. The beam exiting the patient is captured in a digital sensor and the volume reconstructed for viewing in any arbitrary plane. Compared with CBCT, CT images have less noise (ie, they are less grainy), which results from superior collimation of the exit beam in CT machines, thus improving the signal-to-noise ratio but also resulting in greater patient exposure.

CT technology provides a greater range of contrast resolution, displaying soft tissue information not available on CBCT (Fig. 4). CT imaging can be

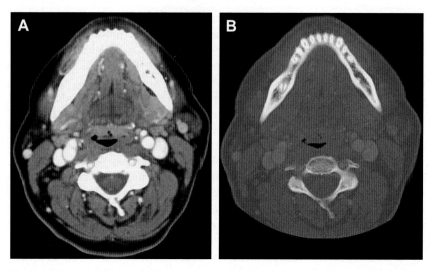

Fig. 4. Soft tissue window. (*A*) CT through mandible in soft tissue window and post administration of iodine. Note sharp definition of muscles in floor of mouth and associated with the
neck. The iodine highlights the great vessels lying just anterior and lateral to cervical vertebrae.
(*B*) Same axial slice displayed in bone window. Note the presence of fine detail in the mandible
and cervical spine, including cortical and cancellous bone, and the teeth, including their pulp
chambers, but the loss of soft tissue contrast. (*From* White SC, Pharoah MJ. Oral radiology,
principles and interpretation. 6th edition. St. Louis (MO): Mosby; in press; with permission.)

improved by the use of intravenous contrast agents, which will enhance the
image contrast of soft tissue entities that have a greater vascularity, such as
tumors. Thus, CT is particularly useful in situations where soft tissue detail
is important, such as when determining whether a tumor arising in bone has
penetrated through the bony cortex and into the adjacent soft tissues. As
with CBCT, CT images may also be presented as 3D solid or translucent
models. In dentistry, 3D CT has been applied to the diagnosis of trauma
and large pathologic conditions, and the assessment of congenital and
acquired skeletal deformities. The DICOM image data are also used to construct life-sized models for trial surgeries, surgical stents for guiding dental
implant placement, and accurate implanted prostheses.

The primary limitation of CT is its high dose compared with cone-beam
examinations. CT examinations are increasingly ordered in medicine and, as
a result, the average person in the United States annually receives as much
radiation from manmade sources as from natural, background sources. Unfortunately, CT also suffers the same metallic artifacts seen in CBCT images.

Clinical considerations

The most frequent indication for CT examinations in dentistry in recent
years has been for evaluating prospective implant sites for the amount and

character of remaining alveolar bone. With the ever-increasing availability of CBCT, many, and perhaps most, such examinations are being made with CBCT machines, which results in a substantial dose savings. However, CT still can provide superior images for some types of pathology, especially where soft tissue information is required. Future clinical experience and research will determine when CT should be used instead of CBCT for the analysis of specific diseases.

MRI

Briefly, to make an MR image, the patient is first placed inside a large magnet [10]. This magnetic field causes the nuclei of many atoms in the body, particularly hydrogen, to align with the magnetic field. The MRI scanner then directs a radiofrequency pulse into the patient, causing some hydrogen nuclei to absorb energy by reversing their orientation (resonate). When the radiofrequency pulse is turned off, the stored energy is released back from the body and detected as a signal in a receiver coil. The stored energy from hydrogen is released with two time constants, T1 and T2 relaxation times. These signals are used to construct the MR images, in essence a map of the distribution of hydrogen. Because soft tissues have a high water content, MRI provides excellent soft tissue contrast resolution. MRI is particularly useful for evaluating soft tissue pathology (Fig. 5). Although x-ray attenuation coefficients of soft tissues may vary by no more than 1%, T1 and T2 relaxation times may vary by up to 40% and are thus readily

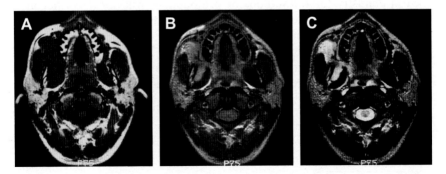

Fig. 5. Gadolinium enhancement of MRI. (*A*) Axial T1 MRI of a rhabdomyosarcoma involving the soft tissues of the right face. The tumor cannot be distinguished from the adjacent masseter and pterygoid muscles because both have the same tissue signal. (*B*) Axial T1 postgadolinium MRI of same case. Note that the tumor now has a brighter signal (lighter) than the adjacent muscles because of its greater vascularity, enhanced by the gadolinium. (*C*) Axial T2 MRI of same case. Note that the tumor has a brighter signal than adjacent muscles because of greater fluid content of the tumor. (*From* White SC, Pharoah MJ. Oral radiology, principles and interpretation. 6th edition. St. Louis (MO): Mosby; in press; with permission.)

distinguished. Like CBCT, MR images may be reconstructed in any imaging plane.

Clinical considerations

MRI examinations are commonly ordered in dentistry to evaluate soft tissue abnormalities of the TMJ, such as the position of the disk in the TMJ. Other indications include evaluating soft tissue disease, especially neoplasia, involving the tongue, cheek, salivary glands, and neck; determining malignant involvement of lymph nodes; and determining perineural invasion by malignant neoplasia. The advantage of MRI is its different and much greater soft tissue contrast resolution compared with X ray–based imaging modalities. The soft tissue contrast of entities that have a greater vascularity can be enhanced with the use of intravenous paramagnetic contrast agents such as gadolinium. A typical diagnostic work-up would include T1, T1 postgadolinium, fat-saturated, and T2-weighted images.

MRI has the distinct advantage of all the imaging modalities discussed in this article of not using ionizing radiation; thus, patient exposure is not a concern. Also, some differences in soft tissue contrast can only be appreciated with MRI; for example, some cases of squamous cell carcinoma of the tongue can only be visualized with MRI. The presence of a strong magnetic field does, however, present the potential of causing movement of ferromagnetic metals in the vicinity of the imaging magnet, which excludes from MRI any patient who has implanted metallic foreign objects or medical devices that consist of, or contain, ferromagnetic metals (eg, cardiac pacemakers, some cerebral aneurysm clips, or ferrous foreign bodies in the eye) because the strong magnetic fields may move these objects and harm patients. Metals used in dentistry for restorations or orthodontics will not move but may distort the image in their vicinity. Titanium implants cause only minor image degradation. Some patients suffer from claustrophobia when positioned in the close confines of an MRI machine. Finally, MRI tends to be expensive. As with other new imaging modalities, specific applications are continually being explored with research and clinical experiences.

Nuclear medicine

Film radiography, CBCT, CT, and MRI, are all morphologic imaging techniques that require a macroscopic anatomic change for information to be recorded. However, abnormal biochemical processes cause some diseases without anatomic changes and, in some cases, the early stage of disease has not allowed enough time for meaningful morphologic changes. Radionuclide imaging is a form of functional imaging that provides a means of assessing such physiologic change in the absence of anatomic change [11,12].

Radionuclide imaging uses radioactive atoms or molecules that emit gamma rays. These atoms behave in an organism in a manner comparable to their stable counterparts because they are chemically indistinguishable. The radionuclide is combined with a pharmaceutic (radiopharmaceutic) that directs the whole molecule to specific parts of the body. After the radiopharmaceutic is administered, the molecules distribute in the body according to their chemical properties. Gamma scintillation cameras detect the gamma rays and form either planar images, image slices similar to CT (single-photon emission computed tomography [SPECT]), or 3D images, all showing the locations of the radionuclides in the body. Radionuclides thus may allow measurement of tissue function in vivo and may provide an early marker of disease through measurement of biochemical change.

The ideal radionuclide has a short half-life, emits gamma rays but no charged particles, and is capable of binding to various pharmaceutics. The most commonly used gamma-emitting isotope is technetium 99m (^{99m}Tc), which has a half-life of 6 hours and emits primarily 140 keV photons. ^{99m}Tc mimics iodine distribution when injected intravenously and is concentrated by the salivary and thyroid glands and gastric mucosa. When it is attached to various carrier molecules, it can be used to examine virtually every organ of the body. The most common use in maxillofacial imaging is the bone scan, which measures bone activity. To image bone, ^{99m}Tc is typically bound to methylene diphosphonate and injected intravenously. The methylene diphosphonate deposits in the skeleton in sites having high osteoblastic activity and in sites having high vascularity. Unfortunately, this method is nonspecific and will be positive for many abnormalities that increase bone metabolism, such as osteomyelitis, osteoarthritis, tumors that either form bone or cause a bone reaction, or areas of active bone growth. Applications include the assessment of condylar growth activity in cases of condylar hyperplasia, abnormal bone activity in occult disease of the jaws, and detection of osteoblastic metastatic tumors involving bone.

Positron emission tomography (PET) is a new technique used to detect abnormally high cellular metabolic rates that may be seen in tumors including metastasis and in inflammatory disease. The usefulness of PET is based not only on its sensitivity but also on the fact that the most commonly used radionuclides (^{11}C, ^{13}N, ^{15}O, ^{18}F) are isotopes of elements that occur naturally in organic molecules. Although fluorine does not technically fit into this category, it is a chemical substitute for hydrogen. These radionuclides are commonly incorporated into a radiopharmaceutic such as glucose or amino acids. After injecting the radiopharmaceutic into the patient, the isotope distributes within the body's tissue according to the carrier molecule, usually to areas of high cellular metabolic activity, and emits a positron that is detected by the PET scanner. PET images are often fused with CT scans to facilitate anatomic localization of radionuclide (Fig. 6). The PET/CT combination has been shown to be helpful in staging and treatment planning of squamous cell carcinoma in the head and neck.

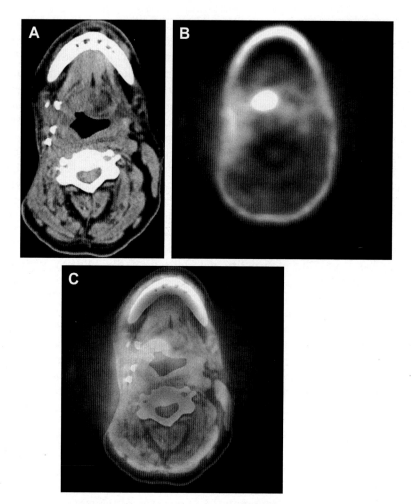

Fig. 6. PET scan and fused PET/CT. This patient has a known recurrent carcinoma at the base of the tongue. (*A*) Soft tissue algorithm CT at level of inferior border of mandible. The four metallic objects on the patient's right side posterior to the mandible represent vascular clips from prior surgery. (*B*) 2-[18F] fluoro-2-deoxy-D-glucose (FDG) PET scan showing oval-shaped region of high metabolic activity of tumor at the right tongue base. The FDG activity in the anterior mandible is related to low-level metabolic activity in the vicinity of a reconstruction plate. (*C*) Fused images *A* and *B* demonstrating the region of high metabolic activity superimposed on the CT anatomy. Images acquired on combined PET/CT scanner. (*Courtesy of* Todd W. Stultz, MD, Cleveland, Ohio.)

References

[1] van der Stelt PF. Filmless imaging: the uses of digital radiography in dental practice. J Am Dent Assoc 2005;136(10):1379–87.

[2] American Dental Association Council on Scientific Affairs. The use of dental radiographs: update and recommendations. J Am Dent Assoc 2006;137:1304–12.

[3] Ludlow JB, Davies-Ludlow LE, Brooks SL, et al. Dosimetry of 3 CBCT devices for oral and maxillofacial radiology: CB Mercuray, NewTom 3G and i-CAT. Dentomaxillofac Radiol 2006;35(4):219–26.

[4] Lofthag-Hansen S, Huumonen S, Gröndahl K, et al. Limited cone-beam CT and intraoral radiography for the diagnosis of periapical pathology. Oral Surg Oral Med Oral Pathol Oral Radiol Endod 2007;103(1):114–9.

[5] Cotton TP, Geisler TM, Holden DT, et al. Endodontic applications of cone-beam volumetric tomography. J Endod 2007;33(9):1121–32.

[6] White SC. Cone-beam imaging in dentistry. Health Physics, in press.

[7] American Dental Association Council on Scientific Affairs. The use of dental radiographs: update and recommendations. J Am Dent Assoc 2006;137(9):1304–12.

[8] Wolbarst AB. Physics of radiology. 2nd edition. Madison (WI): Medical Physics Publishing; 2005.

[9] Bushberg JT, Seibert JA, Leidholdt EM Jr, et al. The essential physics of medical imaging. 2nd edition. Philadelphia: Lippincott Williams & Wilkins; 2002.

[10] Westbrook C, Roth CK, Talbot J. MRI in practice. 3rd edition. Oxford (UK): Blackwell Publishing Ltd.; 2005.

[11] Mettler FA, Guiberteau MJ. Essentials of nuclear medicine. 5th edition. Philadelphia: WB Saunders Co.; 2006.

[12] Sharp PF, Gemmell HG, Murray AD. Practical nuclear medicine. 3rd edition. London: Springer-Verlag; 2005.

ELSEVIER
SAUNDERS

Dent Clin N Am 52 (2008) 707–730

THE DENTAL
CLINICS
OF NORTH AMERICA

What is Cone-Beam CT and How Does it Work?

William C. Scarfe, BDS, FRACDS, MS[a],[*],
Allan G. Farman, BDS, PhD, DSc, MBA[b]

[a]Department of Surgical/Hospital Dentistry, University of Louisville School
of Dentistry, Room 222G, 501 South Preston Street, Louisville, KY 40292, USA
[b]Department of Surgical/Hospital Dentistry, University of Louisville School
of Dentistry, Room 222C, 501 South Preston Street, Louisville, KY 40292, USA

Imaging is an important diagnostic adjunct to the clinical assessment of the dental patient. The introduction of panoramic radiography in the 1960s and its widespread adoption throughout the 1970s and 1980s heralded major progress in dental radiology, providing clinicians with a single comprehensive image of jaws and maxillofacial structures. However, intraoral and extraoral procedures, used individually or in combination, suffer from the same inherent limitations of all planar two-dimensional (2D) projections: magnification, distortion, superimposition, and misrepresentation of structures. Numerous efforts have been made toward three-dimensional (3D) radiographic imaging (eg, stereoscopy, tuned aperture CT) and although CT has been available, its application in dentistry has been limited because of cost, access, and dose considerations. The introduction of cone-beam computed tomography (CBCT) specifically dedicated to imaging the maxillofacial region heralds a true paradigm shift from a 2D to a 3D approach to data acquisition and image reconstruction. Interest in CBCT from all fields of dentistry is unprecedented because it has created a revolution in maxillofacial imaging, facilitating the transition of dental diagnosis from 2D to 3D images and expanding the role of imaging from diagnosis to image guidance of operative and surgical procedures by way of third-party applications software.

* Corresponding author.
E-mail address: wcscar01@gwise.louisville.edu (W.C. Scarfe).

0011-8532/08/$ - see front matter © 2008 Elsevier Inc. All rights reserved.
doi:10.1016/j.cden.2008.05.005

The purpose of this article is to provide an overview of this CBCT technology and an understanding of the influence of technical parameters on image quality and resultant patient radiation exposure.

Background

CBCT is a recent technology. Imaging is accomplished by using a rotating gantry to which an x-ray source and detector are fixed. A divergent pyramidal- or cone-shaped source of ionizing radiation is directed through the middle of the area of interest onto an area x-ray detector on the opposite side. The x-ray source and detector rotate around a rotation fulcrum fixed within the center of the region of interest. During the rotation, multiple (from 150 to more than 600) sequential planar projection images of the field of view (FOV) are acquired in a complete, or sometimes partial, arc. This procedure varies from a traditional medical CT, which uses a fan-shaped x-ray beam in a helical progression to acquire individual image slices of the FOV and then stacks the slices to obtain a 3D representation. Each slice requires a separate scan and separate 2D reconstruction. Because CBCT exposure incorporates the entire FOV, only one rotational sequence of the gantry is necessary to acquire enough data for image reconstruction (Fig. 1).

CBCT was initially developed for angiography [1], but more recent medical applications have included radiotherapy guidance [2] and mammography [3]. The cone-beam geometry was developed as an alternative to conventional CT using either fan-beam or spiral-scan geometries, to provide more rapid acquisition of a data set of the entire FOV and it uses a comparatively less expensive radiation detector. Obvious advantages of such a system, which provides a shorter examination time, include the reduction of image unsharpness caused by the translation of the patient, reduced image distortion due to internal patient movements, and increased x-ray tube efficiency. However, its main disadvantage, especially with larger FOVs, is a limitation in image quality related to noise and contrast resolution because of the detection of large amounts of scattered radiation.

It has only been since the late 1990s that computers capable of computational complexity and x-ray tubes capable of continuous exposure have enabled clinical systems to be manufactured that are inexpensive and small enough to be used in the dental office. Two additional factors have converged to make CBCT possible.

Development of compact high-quality two-dimensional detector arrays

The demands on any x-ray detector in clinical CBCT are hard to fulfill. The detector must be able to record x-ray photons, read off and send the signal to the computer, and be ready for the next acquisition many hundreds of times within a single rotation. Rotation is usually performed within times equivalent to, or less than, panoramic radiography (10–30 seconds), which

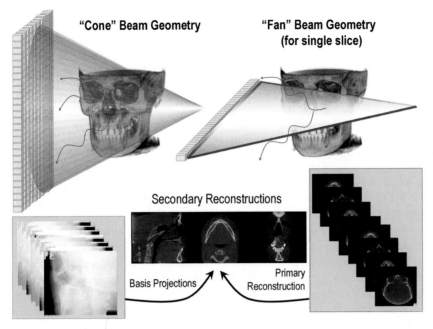

Fig. 1. X-ray beam projection scheme comparing acquisition geometry of conventional or "fan" beam (*right*) and "cone" beam (*left*) imaging geometry and resultant image production. In cone-beam geometry (*left*), multiple basis projections form the projection data from which orthogonal planar images are secondarily reconstructed. In fan beam geometry, primary reconstruction of data produces axial slices from which secondary reconstruction generates orthogonal images. The amount of scatter generated (sinusoidal lines) and recorded by cone-beam image acquisition is substantially higher, reducing image contrast and increasing image noise.

necessitates frame rate image acquisition times of milliseconds. Detectors were initially produced using a configuration of scintillation screens, image intensifiers, and charge-coupled device (CCD) detectors. However, image intensifier systems are large and bulky and FOVs may suffer from peripheral truncation effects (volumetric "cone cuts"), having circular entrance areas rather than more appropriate rectangular ones. Furthermore, rotation of the source-to-detector arrangement may influence sensitivity because of the interference between the magnetic field of the earth and those in the image intensifiers. More recently, high-resolution, inexpensive flat-panel detectors have become available. Such flat detectors are composed of a large-area pixel array of hydrogenated amorphous silicon thin-film transistors. X rays are detected indirectly by means of a scintillator, such as terbium-activated gadolinium oxysulphide or thallium-doped cesium iodide, which converts X rays into visible light that is subsequently registered in the photo diode array. The configuration of such detectors is less complicated and offers greater dynamic range and reduced peripheral distortion; however, these detectors require a slightly greater radiation exposure.

Refinement of approximate cone-beam algorithms

Reconstructing 3D objects from cone-beam projections is a fairly recent accomplishment. In conventional fan-beam CT, individual axial slices of the object are sequentially reconstructed using a well-known mathematic technique (filtered back projection) and subsequently assembled to construct the volume. However, with 2D x-ray area detectors and cone-beam geometry, a 3D volume must be reconstructed from 2D projection data, which is referred to as "cone-beam reconstruction." The first and most popular approximate reconstruction scheme for cone-beam projections acquired along a circular trajectory is the algorithm according to Feldkamp and colleagues [4], referred to as the Feldkamp, Davis, and Kress (FDK) method. This algorithm, used by most research groups and commercial vendors for CBCT with 2D detectors, uses a convolution-back projection method. Although it can be implemented easily with currently available hardware and is a good reconstruction for images at the center or "midplane" of the cone beam, it provides an approximation that causes some unavoidable distortion in the noncentral transverse planes, and resolution degradation in the longitudinal direction. To address this deficiency, several other approaches have been proposed using different algorithms [5] and cone-beam geometries (eg, dual orthogonal circles, helical orbit, orthogonal circle-and-line), and these will no doubt be incorporated into future CBCT designs.

Cone-beam CT image production

Current cone-beam machines scan patients in three possible positions: (1) sitting, (2) standing, and (3) supine. Equipment that requires the patient to lie supine physically occupies a larger surface area or physical footprint and may not be accessible for patients with physical disabilities. Standing units may not be able to be adjusted to a height to accommodate wheelchair-bound patients. Seated units are the most comfortable; however, fixed seats may not allow scanning of physically disabled or wheelchair-bound patients. Because scan times are often greater than those required for panoramic imaging, perhaps more important than patient orientation is the head restraint mechanism used. Despite patient orientation within the equipment, the principles of image production remain the same.

The four components of CBCT image production are (1) acquisition configuration, (2) image detection, (3) image reconstruction, and (4) image display. The image generation and detection specifications of currently available systems (Table 1) reflect proprietary variations in these parameters.

Acquisition configuration

The geometric configuration and acquisition mechanics for the cone-beam technique are theoretically simple. A single partial or full rotational

Table 1
Selected CBCT imaging systems.

Unit	Model(s)	Manufacture/distributor
Accuitomo	3D Accuitomo - XYZ Slice View Tomograph/ Veraviewpacs 3D	J. Morita Mfg. Corp., Kyoto, Japan
Galileos	—	Sirona Dental Systems, Charlotte, North Carolina
Hitachi	CB MercuRay/CB Throne	Hitachi Medical Systems, Tokyo, Japan
i-CAT	Classic/Next Generation	Imaging Sciences International, Hatfield, Pennsylvania
ILUMA	Ultra Cone Beam CT Scanner	IMTEC Imaging, Ardmore, Oklahoma; distributed by KODAK Dental Systems, Carestream Health, Rochester, New York
KaVo	3D eXam	KaVo Dental Corp., Biberach, Germany
KODAK	9000 3D	KODAK Dental Systems, Carestream Health, Rochester, New York
NewTom	3G/NewTom VG	QR, Inc., Verona, Italy/Dent-X Visionary Imaging, Elmsford, New York
Picasso Series	Trio/Pro/Master	E-Woo Technology Co., Ltd./Vatech, Giheung-gu, Korea
PreXion 3D		TeraRecon Inc., San Mateo, California
Promax	3D	Planmeca OY, Helsinki, FInland
Scanora	3D Dental conebeam	SOREDEX, Helsinki, Finland
SkyView	3D Panoramic imager	My-Ray Dental Imaging, Imola, Italy

scan from an x-ray source takes place while a reciprocating area detector moves synchronously with the scan around a fixed fulcrum within the patient's head.

X ray generation

During the scan rotation, each projection image is made by sequential, single-image capture of attenuated x-ray beams by the detector. Technically, the easiest method of exposing the patient is to use a constant beam of radiation during the rotation and allow the x-ray detector to sample the attenuated beam in its trajectory. However, continuous radiation emission does not contribute to the formation of the image and results in greater radiation exposure to the patient. Alternately, the x-ray beam may be pulsed to coincide with the detector sampling, which means that actual exposure time is markedly less than scanning time. This technique reduces patient radiation dose considerably. Currently, four units (Accuitomo, CB Mercu-Ray, Iluma Ultra Cone, and PreXion 3D) provide continuous radiation exposure. Pulsed x-ray beam exposure is a major reason for considerable variation in reported cone-beam unit dosimetry.

Field of view

The dimensions of the FOV or scan volume able to be covered depend primarily on the detector size and shape, the beam projection geometry, and the ability to collimate the beam. The shape of the scan volume can be either cylindric or spherical (eg, NewTom 3G). Collimation of the primary x-ray beam limits x-radiation exposure to the region of interest. Field size limitation therefore ensures that an optimal FOV can be selected for each patient, based on disease presentation and the region designated to be imaged. CBCT systems can be categorized according to the available FOV or selected scan volume height as follows:

Localized region: approximately 5 cm or less (eg, dentoalveolar, temporomandibular joint)
Single arch: 5 cm to 7 cm (eg, maxilla or mandible)
Interarch: 7 cm to 10 cm (eg, mandible and superiorly to include the inferior concha)
Maxillofacial: 10 cm to 15 cm (eg, mandible and extending to Nasion)
Craniofacial: greater than 15 cm (eg, from the lower border of the mandible to the vertex of the head)

Extended FOV scanning incorporating the craniofacial region is difficult to incorporate into cone-beam design because of the high cost of large-area detectors. The expansion of scan volume height has been accomplished by one unit (iCAT Extended Field of View model) by the software addition of two rotational scans to produce a single volume with a 22-cm height. Another novel method for increasing the width of the FOV while using a smaller area detector, thereby reducing manufacturing costs, is to offset the position of the detector, collimate the beam asymmetrically, and scan only half the patient (eg, Scanora 3D, SOREDEX, Helsinki, Finland) (Fig. 2).

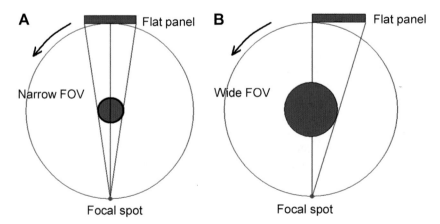

Fig. 2. Novel method of acquiring an extended FOV using a flat panel detector. (*A*) Conventional geometric arrangement whereby the central ray of the x-ray beam from the focal source is directed through the middle of the object to the center of the flat panel detector. (*B*) Alternate method of shifting the location of the flat panel imager and collimating the x-ray beam laterally to extend the FOV object. (*Courtesy of* SOREDEX, Helsinki, Finland; with permission.)

Scan factors

During the scan, single exposures are made at certain degree intervals, providing individual 2D projection images, known as "basis," "frame," or "raw" images. These images are similar to lateral and posterior-anterior "cephalometric" radiographic images, each slightly offset from one another. The complete series of images is referred to as the "projection data." The number of images comprising the projection data throughout the scan is determined by the frame rate (number of images acquired per second), the completeness of the trajectory arc, and the speed of the rotation. The number of projection scans comprising a single scan may be fixed (eg, NewTom 3G, Iluma, Galileos, or Promax 3D) or variable (eg, i-CAT, PreXion 3D). More projection data provide more information to reconstruct the image; allow for greater spatial and contrast resolution; increase the signal-to-noise ratio, producing "smoother" images; and reduce metallic artifacts. However, more projection data usually necessitate a longer scan time, a higher patient dose, and longer primary reconstruction time. In accordance with the "as low as reasonably achievable" (ALARA) principle, the number of basis images should be minimized to produce an image of diagnostic quality.

Frame rate and speed of rotation. Higher frame rates provide images with fewer artifacts and better image quality [6]. However, the greater number of projections proportionately increases the amount of radiation a patient receives. Detector pixels must be sensitive enough to capture radiation adequate to register a high signal-to-noise output and to transmit the voltage to the analog and the digital converter, all within a short arc of exposure. Within the limitations of solid-state detector readout speed and the need of short scanning time in a clinical setting, the total number of available view angles is normally limited to several hundred.

Completeness of the trajectory arc. Most CBCT imaging systems use a complete circular trajectory or a scan arc of 360° to acquire projection data. This physical requirement is usually necessary to produce projection data adequate for 3D reconstruction using the FDK algorithm (see section on reconstruction). However, it is theoretically possible to reduce the completeness of the scanning trajectory and still reconstruct a volumetric data set. This approach potentially reduces the scan time and is mechanically easier to perform. However, images produced by this method may have greater noise and suffer from reconstruction interpolation artifacts. Currently, this technique is used by at least two units (Galileos and Promax 3D).

Image detection

Current CBCT units can be divided into two groups, based on detector type: an image intensifier tube/charge-coupled device (IIT/CCD) combination or a flat-panel imager.

The IIT/CCD configuration comprises an x-ray IIT coupled to a CCD by way of a fiber optic coupling. Flat-panel imaging consists of detection of X rays using an "indirect" detector based on a large-area solid-state sensor panel coupled to an x-ray scintillator layer. Flat-panel detector arrays provide a greater dynamic range and greater performance than the II/CCD technology. Image intensifiers may create geometric distortions that must be addressed in the data processing software, whereas flat-panel detectors do not suffer from this problem. This disadvantage could potentially reduce the measurement accuracy of CBCT units using this configuration. II/CCD systems also introduce additional artifacts [7].

CBCT systems that use flat-panel detectors also have limitations in their performance that are related to linearity of response to the radiation spectrum, uniformity of response throughout the area of the detector, and bad pixels. The effects of these limitations on image quality are most noticeable at lower and higher exposures. To overcome this problem, detectors are linearized piecewise and exposures that cause nonuniformity are identified and calibrated. In addition, pixel-by-pixel standard deviation assessment is used in correcting nonuniformity. Bad pixels are also examined and most often replaced by the average of the neighboring pixels.

A reduction in image matrix size is desirable to increase spatial resolution and therefore provide greater image detail. However, detector panels comprise an array of individual pixels with two components, photodiodes that actually record the image and thin-film transistors that act as collators and carriers of signal information. Therefore, not all of the area of an imager is taken up by the photodiode. In fact, the percentage area of the detector that actually registers information within an individual pixel is referred to as "fill factor." So although a pixel may have a nominal area, the fill factor may be of the order of 35%. Therefore, smaller pixels capture fewer x-ray photons and result in more image noise. Consequently, CBCT imaging using smaller matrix sizes usually requires greater radiation and higher patient dose exposure.

The resolution, and therefore detail, of CBCT imaging is determined by the individual volume elements or voxels produced from the volumetric data set. In CBCT imaging, voxel dimensions primarily depend on the pixel size on the area detector, unlike those in conventional CT, which depend on slice thickness. The resolution of the area detector is submillimeter (range: 0.09 mm to 0.4 mm), which principally determines the size of the voxels. Therefore, CBCT units, in general, provide voxel resolutions that are isotropic (equal in all three dimensions) (Fig. 3).

Image reconstruction

Once the basis projection frames have been acquired, data must be processed to create the volumetric data set. This process is called reconstruction. The number of individual projection frames may be from 100 to

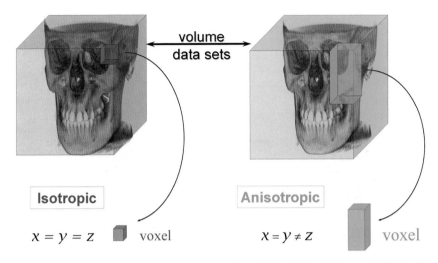

Fig. 3. Comparison of volume data sets obtained isotropically (*left*) and anisotropically (*right*). Because CBCT data acquisition depends on the pixel size of the area detector and not on the acquisition of groups of rows with sequential translational motion, the compositional voxels are equal in all three dimensions, rather than columnar with height being different from the width and depth dimensions.

more than 600, each with more than one million pixels, with 12 to 16 bits of data assigned to each pixel. The reconstruction of the data is therefore computationally complex. To facilitate data handling, data are usually acquired by one computer (acquisition computer) and transferred by way of an Ethernet connection to a processing computer (workstation). In contrast to conventional CT, cone-beam data reconstruction is performed by personal computer rather than workstation platforms.

Reconstruction times vary, depending on the acquisition parameters (voxel size, FOV, number of projections), hardware (processing speed, data throughput from acquisition to workstation computer), and software (reconstruction algorithms) used. Reconstruction should be accomplished in an acceptable time (less than 3 minutes for standard resolution scans) to complement patient flow.

The reconstruction process consists of two stages, each composed of numerous steps (Fig. 4).

Acquisition stage

Because of the spatially varying physical properties of the photodiodes and the switching elements in the flat panel, and also because of variations in the x-ray sensitivity of the scintillator layer, raw images from CBCT detectors show spatial variations of dark image offset and pixel gain. The dark image offset (ie, the detector output signal without any x-ray exposure), and its spatial variations are mainly caused by the varying dark current of the photodiodes. Gain variations are caused by the varying sensitivity of the photodiodes

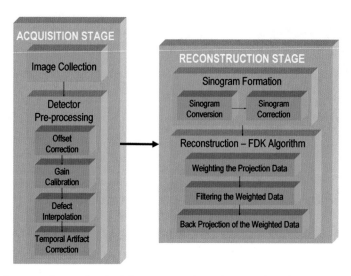

Fig. 4. Stages and steps involved in reconstruction of acquired projection data to form volumetric data from CBCT acquisition. The acquisition stage involves image collection and detector preprocessing, whereas the reconstruction stage involves sinogram formation and reconstruction using the FDK algorithm.

and by variations in the local conversion efficiency of the scintillator material caused by, for example, thickness or density variations. In addition to offset and gain variations, even high-quality detectors exhibit inherent pixel imperfections or a certain amount of defect pixels. To compensate for these inhomogeneities, raw images require systematic offset and gain calibration and a correction of defect pixels. The sequence of the required calibration steps is referred to as "detector preprocessing" (Fig. 5) and the calibration requires the acquisition of additional image sequences [8].

Reconstruction stage

Once images are corrected, they must be related to each other and assembled. One method involves constructing a sinogram: a composite image relating each row of each projection image (Fig. 6). The final step in the reconstruction stage is processing the corrected sinograms. A reconstruction filter algorithm is applied to the sinogram and converts it into a complete 2D CT slice. The most widely used filtered back projection algorithm for cone-beam–acquired volumetric data is the FDK algorithm [4]. Once all the slices have been reconstructed, they can be recombined into a single volume for visualization.

Image display

The availability of CBCT technology provides the dental clinician with a great choice of image display formats. The volumetric data set is

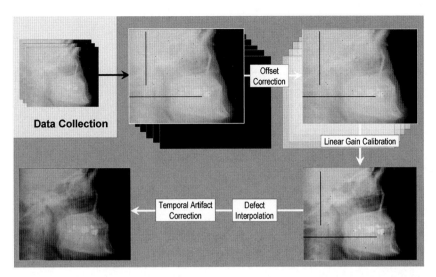

Fig. 5. CBCT detector preprocessing. The first step of the detector preprocessing is the offset correction, which is performed by pixel-wise subtraction of an individual offset value computed by averaging over a series of up to 30 dark images. The second step is the linear gain calibration, consisting of dividing each pixel by its individual gain factor. The gain factors are obtained by averaging a sequence, again with up to 30 images, of homogeneous exposures without any object between x-ray source and detector. The gain sequence is first offset corrected with its own sequence of dark images. The next procedure is the defect interpolation. Each pixel that shows unusual behavior, either in the gain image or in the average dark sequence, is marked in a defect map. The gray values of pixels classified as defective in this way are computed by linear interpolation along the least gradient descent. Flat detectors usually require an additional procedure to correct for temporal artifacts, which arise in flat detectors because the scintillator and photodiodes exhibit residual signals.

a compilation of all available voxels and, for most CBCT devices, it is presented to the clinician on screen as secondary reconstructed images in three orthogonal planes (axial, sagittal, and coronal), usually at a thickness defaulted to the native resolution (Fig. 7). Optimum visualization of orthogonal reconstructed images depends on the adjustment of window level and window width to favor bone and the application of specific filters.

Advantages of cone-beam CT in dentistry

Being considerably smaller, CBCT equipment has a greatly reduced physical footprint and is approximately one quarter to one fifth the cost of conventional CT. CBCT provides images of highly contrasting structures and is therefore particularly well suited for the imaging of osseous structures of the craniofacial area. The use of CBCT technology in clinical dental practice provides a number of advantages for maxillofacial imaging.

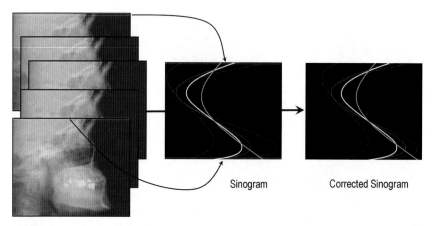

Fig. 6. Construction and correction of sinograms. This process is referred to as the radon transformation. Individual rows of each basis image are extracted and used to develop a composite image. The first row on the first basis image is used to form the first row on the composite image, the first row on the second image is used to form the second row on the composite image, and so on, until the first row on the nth image forms the nth row on the composite image. The resulting image comprises multiple sine waves of different amplitudes. The waves represent features in the object that are being rotated over 360°. However, before reconstruction, sinograms must be corrected for centering errors by detecting the skew in the sinogram and shifting it appropriately. Once corrected, the sinogram is ready to be processed by the appropriate reconstruction algorithm.

Rapid scan time

Because CBCT acquires all projection images in a single rotation, scan time is comparable to panoramic radiography, which is desirable because artifact due to subject movement is reduced. Computer time for data set reconstruction, however, is substantially longer; it varies, depending on FOV, number of basis images acquired, resolution, and reconstruction algorithm, and may range from approximately 1 minute to 20 minutes.

Beam limitation

Collimation of the CBCT primary x-ray beam enables limitation of the x-radiation to the area of interest. Therefore, an optimum FOV can be selected for each patient based on suspected disease presentation and region of interest. Although not available on all CBCT systems, this function is highly desirable because it provides dose savings by limiting the irradiated field to fit the FOV.

Image accuracy

CBCT imaging produces images with submillimeter isotropic voxel resolution ranging from 0.4 mm to as low as 0.076 mm. Because of this

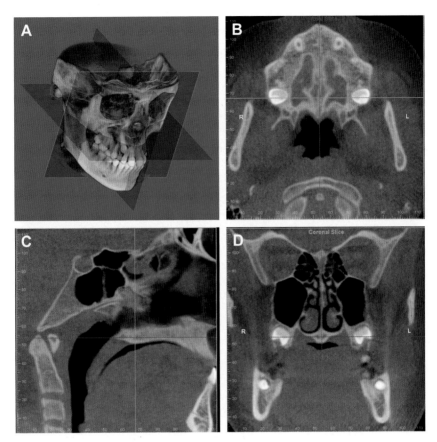

Fig. 7. Standard display modes of CBCT volumetric data. (*A*) Volumetric 3D representation of hard tissue showing the three orthogonal planes in relation to the reconstructed volumetric data set; each orthogonal plane has multiple thin-slice sections in each plane. (*B*) Representative axial image. (*C*) representative sagittal image, and (*D*) representative coronal image. (Images produced using Dolphin 3D, Chatsworth, California).

characteristic, subsequent secondary (axial, coronal, and sagittal) and multiplanar reformation (MPR) images achieve a level of spatial resolution accurate enough for measurement in maxillofacial applications where precision in all dimensions is important, such as implant site assessment and orthodontic analysis.

Reduced patient radiation dose

Published reports indicate that the effective dose [9] varies for various full FOV CBCT devices, ranging from 29 to 477 μSv, depending on the type and model of CBCT equipment and FOV selected (Table 2) [10–12]. Comparing these doses with multiples of a single panoramic dose or background equivalent radiation dose, CBCT provides an equivalent patient radiation dose of

Table 2
Comparative radiation effective dose from selected cone-beam CT systems

CBCT unit	Technique	Dose[a] Absolute Effective dose[a] (μSv)	Comparative Imaging surveys Equivalent panoramic surveys[b]	Annual per capita background[c] No. of days	% Annual
CB MercuRay[d]	12-in/9-in/6-in FOV	477/289/169	74/45/26	48.0/29.0/17.0	13.0/8.0/4.7
Galileos[e]	Default/maximum	29/54	5/9	3.0/5.5	0.8/1.5
i-Cat[d]	12-in/9-in FOV	135/69	21/11	13.5/7.0	3.7/1.9
Iluma[e]	Low/high	61/331	10/53	6.2/33.5	1.7/9.2
Newtom 3G[d]	12-in/9-in FOV	45/37	7/6	4.5/3.5	1.2/1.0
PreXion 3D[e]	Standard/high-resolution	69/160	11/25	7.0/16.0	1.9/4.4
ProMax 3D[e]	Small/large	157/210	25/33	16.0/21.5	4.4/5.8

[a] Using 1990 International Commission on Radiological Protection calculations.
[b] *Data from* Ludlow JB, Davies-Ludlow LE, Brooks SL. Dosimetry of two extraoral direct digital imaging devices: NewTom cone beam CT and Orthophos Plus DS panoramic unit. Dentomaxillofac Radiol 2003;32:229–34.
[c] Annual per capita = 3.6 mSv (3600 μSv) per annum.
[d] *Data from* Ludlow JB, Davies-Ludlow LE, Brooks SL. Dosimetry of 3 CBCT devices for oral and maxillofacial radiology: CB Mercuray, NewTom 3G and i-CAT. Dentomaxillofac Radiol 2006;35:219–26.
[e] *Data from* Ludlow JB, Davies-Ludlow LE, Mol A. Dosimetry of recently introduced CBCT units for oral and maxillofacial radiology. Proceedings of the 16th International Congress of Dentomaxillofacial Radiology. Beijing, China, June 26–30, 2007. p. 97.

5 to 74 times that of a single film-based panoramic X ray, or 3 to 48 days of background radiation. Patient positioning modifications (tilting the chin) and use of additional personal protection (thyroid collar) can substantially reduce the dose by up to 40% [9,10]. Comparison with patient dose reported for maxillofacial imaging by conventional CT (approximately 2000 µSv) indicates that CBCT provides substantial dose reductions of between 98.5% and 76.2% [11–13].

Interactive display modes applicable to maxillofacial imaging

Perhaps the most important advantage of CBCT is that it provides unique images demonstrating features in 3D that intraoral, panoramic, and cephalometric images cannot. CBCT units reconstruct the projection data to provide interrelational images in three orthogonal planes (axial, sagittal, and coronal). In addition, because reconstruction of CBCT data is performed natively using a personal computer, data can be reoriented so that the patient's anatomic features are realigned. Basic enhancements include zoom or magnification, window/level, and the ability to add annotation. Cursor-driven measurement algorithms provide the clinician with an interactive capability for real-time dimensional assessment. On-screen measurements provide dimensions free from distortion and magnification.

Multiplanar reformation

Because of the isotropic nature of the volumetric data sets, they can be sectioned nonorthogonally. Most software provides for various nonaxial 2D images, referred to as MPR. Such MPR modes include oblique, curved planar reformation (providing "simulated" distortion-free panoramic images), and serial transplanar reformation (providing cross-sections), all of which can be used to highlight specific anatomic regions and diagnostic tasks (Fig. 8), which is important, given the complex structure of the maxillofacial region.

Because of the large number of component orthogonal images in each plane and the difficulty in relating adjacent structures, two methods have been developed to visualize adjacent voxels.

Ray sum or ray casting

Any multiplanar image can be "thickened" by increasing the number of adjacent voxels included in the display, which creates an image slab that represents a specific volume of the patient, referred to as a ray sum. Full-thickness perpendicular ray sum images can be used to generate simulated projections such as lateral cephalometric images (Fig. 9). Unlike conventional X rays, these ray sum images are without magnification and are undistorted. However, this technique uses the entire volumetric data set, and interpretation suffers from the problems of "anatomic noise," the superimposition of multiple structures.

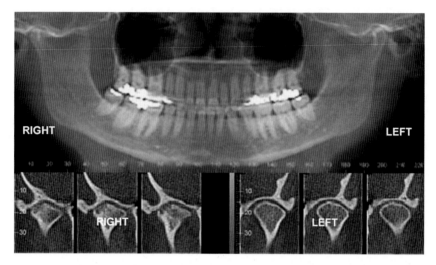

Fig. 8. Curved MPR simulated "panoramic" image from CBCT showing CBCT applications in temporomandibular joint assessment. Reformatted "panoramic" image (*top*) showing right side condyle differences in shape compared with normal left. Cropped paracoronal reformatted images clearly showing subcortical cystic defects in surface of right condyle as compared with the left, indicative of active degenerative joint disease. Images generated using i-CAT (Imaging Sciences International, Hatsfield, Pennsylvania).

Three-dimensional volume rendering

Volume rendering refers to techniques that allow the visualization of 3D data through integration of large volumes of adjacent voxels and selective display (Fig. 10). Two specific techniques are available.

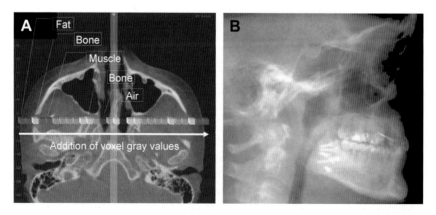

Fig. 9. Construction of ray sum images. An axial projection (*A*) is used as the reference image. A section slice is identified (*dashed line*) which, in this case, corresponds to the midsagittal plane and the thickness of this slice is increased to include the left and right sides of the volumetric data set. As the thickness of the "slab" increases, adjacent voxels representing elements such as air, bone, and soft tissues are added. The resultant image (*B*) generated from a full-thickness ray sum provides a simulated lateral cephalometric image.

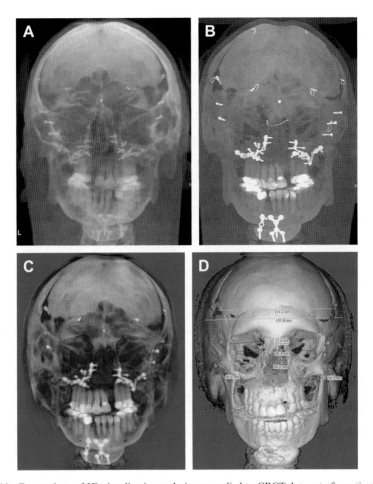

Fig. 10. Comparison of 3D visualization techniques applied to CBCT data set of a patient who has a craniofacial deformity. Anterior-posterior projection rendered using the direct volume rendering techniques of (*A*) ray sum and (*B*) maximum intensity projection and the indirect volume techniques of (*C*) volumetric transparent and (*D*) shaded surface display. Volumetric data set acquired with extended FOV i-CAT (Imaging Sciences International, Hatsfield, Pennsylvania) and all reconstructions generated using Dolphin 3D (Dolphin Imaging, Chatsworth, California).

Indirect volume rendering. Indirect volume rendering is a complex process, requiring selecting the intensity or density of the grayscale level of the voxels to be displayed within an entire data set (called segmentation). This technique is technically demanding and computationally difficult, requiring specific software; however, it provides a volumetric surface reconstruction with depth.

Direct volume rendering. Clinically and technically, direct volume rendering is a much more simple process. The most common direct volume rendering technique is maximum intensity projection (MIP). MIP visualizations are achieved by evaluating each voxel value along an imaginary projection ray from the observer's eyes within a particular volume of interest and then representing only the highest value as the display value. Voxel intensities that are below an arbitrary threshold are eliminated.

Limitations of cone-beam CT imaging

While clinical applications of CBCT have expanded, current CBCT technology has limitations related to the "cone-beam" projection geometry, detector sensitivity, and contrast resolution that produces images that lack the clarity and usefulness of conventional CT images. The clarity of CBCT images is affected by artifacts, noise, and poor soft tissue contrast.

Artifacts

An artifact is any distortion or error in the image that is unrelated to the subject being studied. Artifacts can be classified according to their cause.

X-ray beam artifacts

CT image artifacts arise from the inherent polychromatic nature of the projection x-ray beam that results in what is known as beam hardening (ie, its mean energy increases because lower energy photons are absorbed in preference to higher energy photons). This beam hardening results in two types of artifact: (1) distortion of metallic structures due to differential absorption, known as a cupping artifact, and (2) streaks and dark bands that can appear between two dense objects. Because the CBCT x-ray beam is heterochromatic and has lower mean kilovolt (peak) energy compared with conventional CT, this artifact is more pronounced on CBCT images. In clinical practice, it is advisable to reduce the FOV to avoid scanning regions susceptible to beam hardening (eg, metallic restorations, dental implants), which can be achieved by collimation, modification of patient positioning, or separation of the dental arches. More recently, dental CBCT manufacturers have introduced artifact reduction technique algorithms within the reconstruction process (eg, Scanora 3D, SOREDEX, Helsinki, Finland) (Fig. 11). These algorithms reduce image-, noise-, metal-, and motion-related artifacts and require fewer projection images, and therefore may allow for a lower acquisition dose. However, they are computationally demanding and require increased reconstruction times.

Patient-related artifacts

Patient motion can cause misregistration of data, which appears as unsharpness in the reconstructed image. This unsharpness can be minimized by using a head restraint and as short a scan time as possible. The presence of dental restorations in the FOV can lead to severe streaking artifacts. They

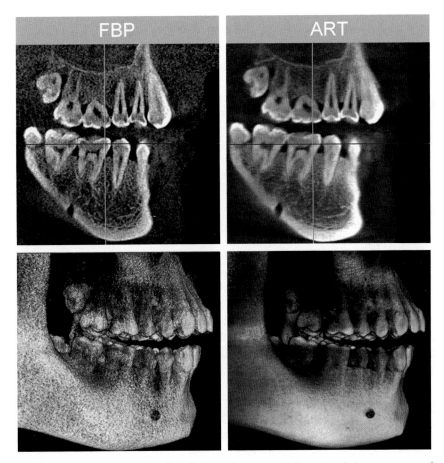

Fig. 11. Comparison of image quality of sagittal (*upper*) and 3D (*lower*) renderings reconstructed from 300 projection images using conventional Feldkamp back projection (FBP) (*left column*) and an iterative reconstruction called algebraic reconstruction technique (ART) (*right column*). While ART requires greater computing power, it also reduces artifacts requiring fewer projections to conduct the reconstruction (equals less dose) and is less sensitive to common patient movement and metal artifacts. (*Courtesy of* SOREDEX, Helsinki, Finland; with permission.)

occur because of extreme beam hardening or photon starvation due to insufficient photons reaching the detector, resulting in horizontal streaks in the image and noisy projection reconstructions. This problem can be reduced by removing metallic objects such as jewelry before scanning commences.

Scanner-related artifacts

Typically, scanner-related artifacts present as circular or ring-shaped, resulting from imperfections in scanner detection or poor calibration. Either of these two problems will result in a consistent and repetitive reading at each angular position of the detector, resulting in a circular artifact.

Cone beam–related artifacts

The beam projection geometry of the CBCT and the image reconstruction method produce three types of cone-beam–related artifacts: (1) partial volume averaging, (2) undersampling, and (3) cone-beam effect.

Partial volume averaging. Partial volume averaging is a feature of conventional fan and CBCT imaging. It occurs when the selected voxel resolution of the scan is greater than the spatial or contrast resolution of the object to be imaged. In this case, the pixel is not representative of the tissue or boundary; however, it becomes a weighted average of the different CT values. Boundaries in the resultant image may present with a "step" appearance or homogeneity of pixel intensity levels. Partial volume averaging artifacts occur in regions where surfaces are rapidly changing in the z direction (eg, in the temporal bone). Selection of the smallest acquisition voxel can reduce the presence of these effects.

Undersampling. Undersampling can occur when too few basis projections are provided for the reconstruction. A reduced data sample leads to misregistration and sharp edges and noisier images because of aliasing, where fine striations appear in the image. This effect may not degrade the image severely; however, when resolution of fine detail is important, undersampling artifacts need to be avoided as far as possible by maintaining the number of basis projection images.

Cone-beam effect. The cone-beam effect is a potential source of artifacts, especially in the peripheral portions of the scan volume. Because of the divergence of the x-ray beam as it rotates around the patient in a horizontal plane, projection data are collected by each detector pixel. The amount of data corresponds to the total amount of recorded attenuation along a specific beam projection angle as the scanner completes an arc (Fig. 12). The total amount of information for peripheral structures is reduced because the outer row detector pixels record less attenuation, whereas more information is recorded for objects projected onto the more central detector pixels, which results in image distortion, streaking artifacts, and greater peripheral noise. This effect is minimized by manufacturers incorporating various forms of cone-beam reconstruction. Clinically, it can be reduced by positioning the region of interest adjacent to the horizontal plane of the x-ray beam and collimation of the beam to an appropriate FOV.

Image noise

The cone-beam projection acquisition geometry results in a large volume being irradiated with every basis image projection. As a result, a large portion of the photons engage in interactions by way of attenuation. Most of these occur by Compton scattering producing scattered radiation.

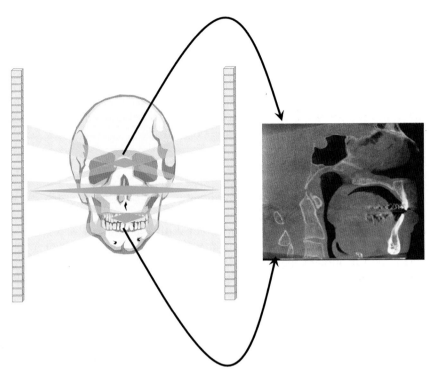

Fig. 12. Origin of the cone-beam effect. The projection of three x-ray beams (one perpendicular, one angled inferiorly, and the other angled superiorly) from a point origin are shown at two positions of the x-ray tube, 180° apart. The amount of data collected by the detector for reconstruction corresponds to the solid volume between the overlapping projections. Centrally, the amount of data acquired is maximal, whereas peripherally, the amount of data collected is appreciably less. The midsagittal section image demonstrates the visual effects of this in producing a peripheral "V" artifact of increased noise, distortion, and reduced contrast.

Most of the scattered radiation is produced omnidirectionally and is recorded by pixels on the cone-beam area detector, which does not reflect the actual attenuation of the object within a specific path of the x-ray beam. This additional recorded x-ray attenuation, reflecting nonlinear attenuation, is called noise. Because of the use of an area detector, much of this nonlinear attenuation is recorded and contributes to image degradation or noise. The scatter-to-primary ratios are about 0.01 for single-ray CT and 0.05 to 0.15 for fan-beam and spiral CT, and may be as large as 0.4 to 2.0 in CBCT. Problems also exist with detectors and algorithms.

Poor soft tissue contrast

Three factors limit the contrast resolution of CBCT. Although scattered radiation contributes to increased image noise, it is also a significant factor in reducing the contrast of the cone-beam system. In addition, the divergence of the x-ray beam over the area detector causes a pronounced heel effect. This effect produces a large variation in, or nonuniformity of, the incident x-ray beam on the patient and resultant nonuniformity in absorption, with greater signal-to-noise ratio (noise) on the cathode side of the image relative to the anode side. Finally, numerous inherent flat-panel detector-based artifacts affect its linearity or response to x-radiation. Although these conditions limit the application of current CBCT imaging to the assessment of osseous structures, several techniques and devices are currently being investigated to suppress this effect.

Applications

Currently, CBCT is used most commonly in the assessment of bony and dental pathologic conditions, including fracture; structural maxillofacial deformity and fracture recognition; preoperative assessment of impacted teeth; and temporomandibular joint imaging; and in the analysis of available bone for implant placement. In orthodontics, CBCT imaging is now being directed toward 3D cephalometry. These applications are described in detail in other articles.

The availability of CBCT is also expanding the use of additional diagnostic and treatment software applications, all directed toward 3D visualization, because CBCT data can be exported in the nonproprietary Digital Imaging and Communications in Medicine file format standard. CBCT permits more than diagnosis; it facilitates image-guided surgery. Diagnostic and planning software are available to assist in orthodontic assessment and analysis (eg, Dolphin 3D, Dolphin Imaging, Chatsworth, California) and in implant planning to fabricate surgical models (eg, Biomedical Modeling Inc., Boston, Massachusetts); to facilitate virtual implant placement; to create diagnostic and surgical implant guidance stents (eg, Virtual Implant Placement, Implant Logic Systems, Cedarhurst, New York; Simplant, Materialise, Leuven, Belgium; EasyGuide, Keystone Dental, Burlington, Massachusetts); and even to assist in the computer-aided design and manufacture of implant prosthetics (NobelGuide/Procera software, Nobel Care AG, Göteborg, Sweden). Software is also available to provide surgical simulations for osteotomies and distraction osteogenesis (Maxilim, Medicim NV, Mechelen, Belgium). This area is a blossoming field that provides opportunities for practitioners to combine CBCT diagnosis and 3D simulations with virtual surgery and computer-assisted design and manufacture. Image guidance is an exciting advance that will undoubtedly have a substantial impact on dentistry.

Clinical implications

The impact that CBCT technology has had on maxillofacial imaging since its introduction cannot be underestimated, which does not imply that CBCT is appropriate as an imaging modality of first choice in dental practice. However, no specific patient selection criteria have been published for the use of CBCT in maxillofacial imaging (ie, guidelines as to when, where, why, what, how, and on whom). Because cone-beam exposure provides a radiation dose to the patient higher than any other imaging procedure in dentistry, it is paramount that practitioners abide by the ALARA principle. The basis of this principle is that the justification of the exposure to the patient is that the total potential diagnostic benefits are greater than the individual detriment radiation exposure might cause. CBCT should not be considered a replacement for standard digital radiographic applications that, ironically, also use a cone beam of radiation, but without computed integration of basis projections. Rather, CBCT is a complementary modality for specific applications.

Although deceptively simple, the technical component of patient exposure is only one half of cone-beam imaging. Based on the medical model of imaging, a moral, ethical, and legal responsibility of interpreting the resultant volumetric data set exists [14–16]. The mechanics of interpretation involve image reporting with the development of a series of images formatted to display the condition/region appropriately (image report) and a cognitive interpretation of the significance of the imaging findings (interpretive report). These skills are not within the domain of most general and specialist practitioners; however, they act as the de facto standard of care in providing CBCT services. It would behoove those contemplating or currently using CBCT imaging to develop and maintain these skills.

Summary

The development and rapid commercialization of CBCT technology dedicated for use in the maxillofacial region will undoubtedly increase general and specialist practitioner access to this imaging modality. CBCT is capable of providing accurate, submillimeter-resolution images in formats allowing 3D visualization of the complexity of the maxillofacial region. All current generations of CBCT systems provide useful diagnostic images. Future enhancements will most likely be directed toward reducing scan time; providing multimodal imaging (conventional panoramic and cephalometric, in addition to CBCT images); improving image fidelity, including soft tissue contrast; and incorporating task-specific protocols to minimize patient dose (eg, high-resolution, small FOV for dentoalveolar imaging or medium-resolution, large FOV for dentofacial orthopedic imaging). The increasing availability of this technology provides the practitioner with a modality that is extending maxillofacial imaging from diagnosis to image guidance of operative and surgical procedures.

References

[1] Robb RA. Dynamic spatial reconstruction: an x-ray video fluoroscopic CT scanner for dynamic volume imaging of moving organs. IEEE Trans Med Imag 1982;M1:22–3.

[2] Cho PS, Johnson RH, Griffin TW. Cone-beam CT for radiotherapy applications. Phys Med Biol 1995;40:1863–83.

[3] Ning R, Chen B. Cone beam volume CT mammographic imaging: feasibility study. In: Antonuk LE, Yaffe MJ, editors. Medical imaging 2001: physics of medical imaging—proceedings of SPIE. vol. 4320. San Diego (CA): CA SPIE; 2001. p. 655–64.

[4] Feldkamp LA, Davis LC, Kress JW. Practical cone-beam algorithm. J Opt Soc Am 1984; A1(6):612–9.

[5] Wischmann H-A, Luijendijk HA, Meulenbrugge HJ, et al. Correction of amplifier nonlinearity, offset, gain, temporal artifacts, and defects for flat-panel digital imaging devices. In: Antonuk LE, Yaffe MJ, editors. Medical imaging 2002: physics of medical imaging—proceedings of SPIE. vol. 4682. San Diego (CA): CA SPIE; 2002. p. 427–37.

[6] Grangeat P. Mathematical framework of cone beam 3D reconstruction via the first derivate of the Radon transform. In: Herman GT, Luis AK, Natterer F, editors. Mathematical methods in tomography. Volume 1497. Berlin (Germany): Springer Verlag; 1991. p. 66–97.

[7] International Commission on Radiological Protection. 1990 Recommendations of the International Commission on Radiological Protection, ICRP Publication 60. Ann ICRP 1991;21:1–201.

[8] Ludlow JB, Davies-Ludlow LE, Brooks SL. Dosimetry of two extraoral direct digital imaging devices: NewTom cone beam CT and Orthophos Plus DS panoramic unit. Dentomaxillofac Radiol 2003;32:229–34.

[9] Ludlow JB, Davies-Ludlow LE, Brooks SL, et al. Dosimetry of 3 CBCT devices for oral and maxillofacial radiology: CB Mercuray, NewTom 3G and i-CAT. Dentomaxillofac Radiol. 2006;35:219–26 [erratum in: Dentomaxillofac Radiol. 2006;35:392].

[10] Ludlow JB, Davies-Ludlow LE, Mol A. Dosimetry of recently introduced CBCT units for oral and maxillofacial radiology. In: Proceedings of the16th International Congress of Dentomaxillofacial Radiology, Beijing, China 26–30 June, 2007. p. 97.

[11] Schulze D, Heiland M, Thurmann H, et al. Radiation exposure during midfacial imaging using 4- and 16-slice computed tomography, cone beam computed tomography systems and conventional radiography. Dentomaxillofac Radiol 2004;33:83–6.

[12] Scaf G, Lurie AG, Mosier KM, et al. Dosimetry and cost of imaging osseointegrated implants with film-based and computed tomography. Oral Surg Oral Med Oral Pathol Oral Radiol Endod 1997;83:41–8.

[13] Dula K, Mini R, van der Stelt PF, et al. Hypothetical mortality risk associated with spiral computed tomography of the maxilla and mandible. Eur J Oral Sci 1996;104:503–10.

[14] Holmes SM. iCAT scanning in the oral surgery office. OMS National Insurance Company Newsletter; Rosemont (IL); 2007;18 181.

[15] Turpin DL. Befriend your oral and maxillofacial radiologist. Am J Orthod Dentofacial Orthop 2007;131:697.

[16] Holmes SM. Risk management advice for imaging services in the OMS office. OMS National Insurance Company Newsletter; Rosemont (IL); 2008;19:1–5.

ELSEVIER
SAUNDERS

Dent Clin N Am 52 (2008) 731–752

THE DENTAL
CLINICS
OF NORTH AMERICA

Cone Beam Tomographic Imaging Anatomy of the Maxillofacial Region

Christos Angelopoulos, DDS, MS

*Division of Oral and Maxillofacial Radiology, Columbia University,
College of Dental Medicine, PH-7 Stem-134, New York, NY 10032, USA*

The main challenge in cone beam CT (CBCT) imaging and diagnosis is the lack of familiarity experienced by most dental professionals with the concept of multiplanar imaging that is offered by this new and exciting technology. Dentists and specialists, with only a few exceptions, have a wide experience in diagnosis using the traditional dental imaging modalities (intraoral radiography and panoramic radiography), and the comfort level in their diagnostic skills with these modalities is high. These imaging modalities have been taught for several decades in the dental schools and in other training courses.

Diagnostic imaging in different planes is a new concept and may require a different view of the imaging data. It is reminded that multiplanar imaging or reformatting is the ability to generate images in different planes, flat or curved. This ability is offered only by some contemporary imaging modalities, such as CBCT, medical CT, MRI, ultrasound, and others. Because a volume of data has been acquired and stored by CBCT, these data can be reformatted or realigned and several different types of images can be synthesized in any way the diagnostician requires. With multiplanar imaging, the diagnostician or operator can recreate images in different planes (flat or curved) with simple functions. This increases the diagnostic efficiency in the hands of the knowledgeable individual in an unparalleled way (Fig. 1).

In this article, the author reviews the appearance of several anatomic structures of the maxillofacial region and the head and neck region in general; these structures are revealed in a variety of planes (eg, axial, coronal, sagittal, and more). What may add to the complexity of these images is the fact that this technology may demonstrate structures of interest, such as teeth and jaws, in a view that dental professionals have not seen in the past; dentists were never able to view the third dimension of the regions

E-mail address: ca2291@columbia.edu

0011-8532/08/$ - see front matter © 2008 Elsevier Inc. All rights reserved.
doi:10.1016/j.cden.2008.07.002   *dental.theclinics.com*

A   **B**   **C**

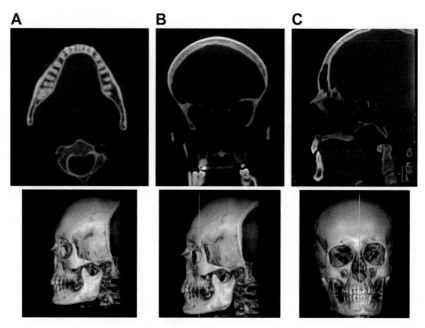

Fig. 1. Multiplanar imaging and reformatting. Axial (*A*), coronal (*B*), and sagittal (*C*) sections of the head. The approximate tomographic plane is shown in the three-dimensional images (*blue line*). These sections can be generated with simple functions using the CBCT scanner's software applications.

of interest. From the beginning, this may make the images look unfamiliar and different.

First, as with every other dental diagnostic image, the images are viewed as if the patient under examination were sitting opposite the dentist, as in the dental chair. The structures identified on the dentist's right side would represent the anatomic structures on the patient's left and vice versa. Most of the available software of the various manufacturers properly identifies the right and left sides or the buccal and lingual sides of the images; thus, orientation is not difficult.

The author starts with the evaluation of well-known dental structures in the maxillofacial region in cross sections. Cross-sectional images are generated perpendicular to the arch-form of the maxilla or mandible. The image demonstrated in Fig. 2 is a cross-sectional image (cut or slice) of the maxilla and mandible in the first molar location. In this image, the buccal and palatal or lingual sides are clearly identified.

The maxillary sinus is a pyramidal in shape low-density (black or dark) structure. The appearance of healthy air cavities in the maxillary sinuses is dark (black) because of the fact that air attenuates x-rays minimally. The thin cortical outline of the buccal and medial sinus walls can be identified in these images. The medial wall of the maxillary sinus borders the sinus

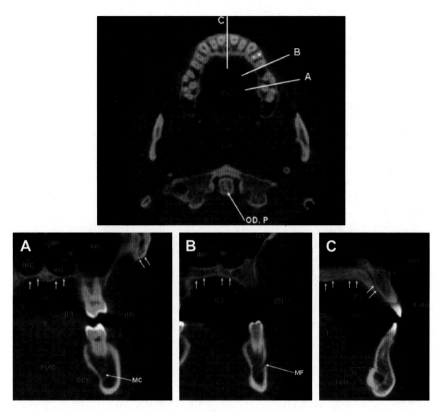

Fig. 2. Axial image (*upper*) at the level of the maxillary alveolar ridge demonstrates the approximate locations of the cross sections A, B, and C. The white lines correspond to the respective sections: odontoid process of axis (ODP) and second cervical vertebra. (*A*) Cross-sectional images in the molar region: the buccal (B), labial (Lab), lingual (L), or palatal (P) aspect of the alveolar bone is marked on the images. FOM, floor of mouth; INC, inferior nasal concha; INF, inferior nasal meatus; MC, mandibular canal; MS, maxillary sinus; OC, oral cavity; SGF, submandibular gland fossa; T, tongue. The green arrows indicate the hard palate, and the yellow arrows indicate the zygomatic process of the maxilla. Note the presence of inflammatory tissue on the floor of the maxillary sinus. The air cavities appear dark (*black*) in CT images. (*B*) Premolar region: MS, maxillary sinus; INC, inferior nasal concha; INF, inferior nasal meatus; OC, oral cavity; T, tongue; FOM, floor of mouth; MF, mental foramen. The green arrows indicate the hard palate. (*C*) Central incisor region: the buccal (B), (Lab), (L), or (P) aspect of the alveolar bone is marked on the images. ANS, anterior nasal spine; OC, oral cavity; T, tongue. The green arrows mark the hard palate, the yellow arrows show the nasopalatine canal, and the red arrows show the lingual foramina (superior and inferior).

cavity from the nasal cavity. Note the soft tissue coverage of the nasal cavity being demonstrated as gray in the image. The high-density core is the inferior nasal concha. The reader is reminded that the inferior nasal concha is an independent facial bone, whereas the rest of the conchae, middle and superior nasal conchae, are parts of the ethmoid bone. Also note that the soft tissue in the region (intraoral and extraoral) demonstrates an almost uniform density; CBCT soft tissue contrast is not adequate to demonstrate differences in musculature or fat, for example.

Further inferior in the same image, you can identify a cross section of the mandibular molar region and the long axis of the mandibular bone in the cross section. Note that the mandibular teeth are not always parallel with the long axis of the mandibular bone in the cross section. The cortical outline of the mandibular bone appears to be much thicker than that of the maxilla (discussed previously). Moreover, the submandibular gland fossa sometimes is more prominent than others. This undercut can be rather severe at times and may impose an anatomic limitation in implant placement in the region. Last, significant anatomic structures, such as the lingual artery, are passing nearby. The mandibular canal is identified into the mandibular bone.

As we move more anteriorly, we are examining cross-sectional images in the premolar locations. You can see similar anatomic structures as the ones before; however, the further anterior we go, the narrower the maxillary sinuses become because we are approaching the anterior wall of the maxillary sinuses. In this cross section, we can see the anterior opening of the mandibular canal, which is the mental foramen. There is considerable variation in the appearance of the mental foramen and its emergence angle (opening angle) into the buccal aspect of the mandibular bone.

The next cross section is along the midline of the maxilla and the mandible, and some different anatomic structures are seen: in this case, the floor of the nasal cavity and the nasopalatine canal. The reader is reminded that the nasopalatine canal starts from the floor of the nasal cavity (inferior meatus) with dual foramina (superior foramina). It carries branches of the nasopalatine nerve, which exit the canal through the incisive foramen and spread to the anterior aspect of the hard palate (see Fig. 2C). The nasopalatine canal may vary in dimensions, and also may pose a limitation in placing implants in this aesthetic zone, the anterior maxilla.

Once more, great variation exists concerning the shape of the anterior mandible in cross sections. A significant anatomic structure in the lingual aspect of the mandibular bone, along the midline of the mandible, is the lingual foramen or foramina, which accommodate the terminal branches of the lingual artery (see Fig. 2C; Fig. 3). Often, they are closely associated with the genial tubercles (high-density structures), which serve as muscle attachment points. The diameter of these canals or foramina is related to the blood-supplying capacity of the blood vessel, and as a result, if they are wide enough, they may bleed significantly if injured during surgical procedures, such as implant surgery [1]. Despite the fact that they are located toward the inferior third of the mandibular bone, they may be seen closer to the crest pending atrophy of the anterior alveolar ridge.

Additional vascular canals are noted from time to time in the mandibular bone anterior to the premolar locations in a region that generally is considered to be a safe site for implant placement (interforaminal region). These

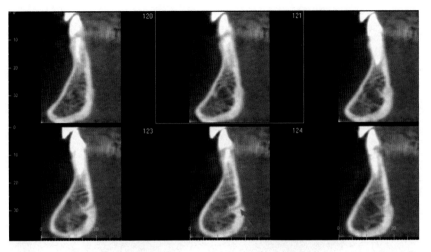

Fig. 3. A series of cross-sectional images in the mandibular central incisor region. The narrow opening in the lingual mandibular cortex (*red arrow*) is the lingual foramen, a vascular canal along the midline, through which the terminal branches of the lingual artery enter the mandibular bone. This canal has been reported as a concern for significant bleeding (pending on its diameter) if punctured during implant surgery.

canals often represent accessory lingual foramina that host accessory branches of the lingual artery. Depending on the width, they may also pose limitations for surgical procedures [2]. Once more, these foramina are identified fairly inferior, unless severe bone resorption is noted (Fig. 4).

The variation of the shape and size of the alveolar ridge is remarkable. After tooth extraction, the maxillary bone and mandibular bone rarely remain unchanged. Frequently, the edentulous areas are accompanied by undercuts as a result of bone resorption, and these undercuts may pose anatomic limitations in implant placement in the posterior mandible (Figs. 5 and 6).

The reader has now become familiar with the cross-sectional imaging of the major anatomic structures in the oral cavity that the dentist frequently uses and identifies in routine dental radiographs. The author now examines these anatomic structures among others in different planes: axial, coronal, and sagittal planes. Once more, these images are reviewed as if the patient were opposite the dentist. Consequently, the right side of the patient's face or the right anatomic structures are on the dentist's left and vice versa. Axial sections (cuts) are the images that have been generated perpendicular to the long axis of the human body (the long axis of the head in this case). These images section the teeth perpendicular to their long axis; as a result, the dentist is able to see transverse sections of the roots and crowns of the teeth in the areas of interest.

Axial images are excellent for the evaluation of the visible parts of the neck and cervical spine, integrity of the palatal and buccal cortical plates

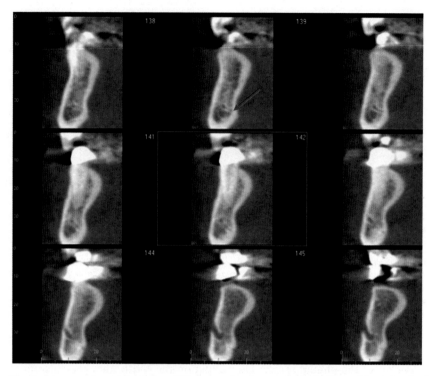

Fig. 4. Accessory lingual foramina. Although not as frequently as the lingual foramina (*red arrow*) noted along the midline of the mandible, additional vascular channels may be present anterior to the premolar locations unilaterally or bilaterally. Depending on their diameter, they may pose a similar limitation to implant surgery as their midline counterparts.

of the maxillary and mandibular dentition, lateral and medial wall of the sinuses, lateral walls of the nasal cavity, anatomic structures in the nasal cavity, zygomatic bones and zygomatic arches, and skull base, for example.

Only parts of the patient's neck can be visualized toward the inferior end of the imaging volume. Soft tissue structures are mostly present at that level (Fig. 7). The inferior border of the anterior mandible may be sectioned at this level and may be visualized toward the superior border of the image. The hyoid bone and the body and the processes of the C3 to C4 vertebrae are expected to be seen in the same cuts. The soft tissue structures identified in this image include the sternocleidomastoid muscles bilaterally, the genio-hyoid muscles, and the submandibular salivary glands. In the center of the image, this semicircular low-density (dark structure) in the middle of the image represents the patient's airway. The airway is separated almost in two halves by a soft tissue structure that is crescent in shape (and some times irregular in appearance), the epiglottis. Approximately at this level, the common carotid artery bifurcates into two main branches, the internal carotid and external carotid arteries, which supply the brain and face of each

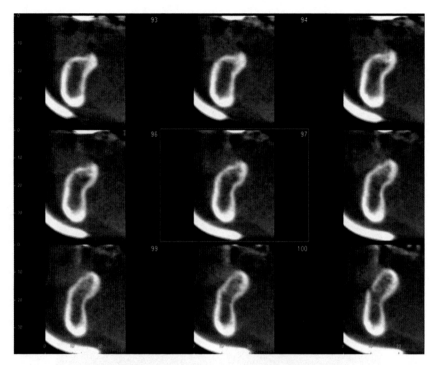

Fig. 5. Alveolar ridge variation. A series of cross-sectional cuts in the mandibular premolar and molar areas shows a marked lingual inclination of the tooth-bearing part of the alveolar bone. Moreover, a lingual undercut is noted extending to the premolar regions (*lower three cross sections*).

side, respectively. The most reliable reported landmarks to indicate the level at which bifurcation occurs are the C3 and C4 levels and the superior border of the thyroid cartilage of the larynx; however, variation is not uncommon (see Fig. 7; Fig. 8). Superior to the bifurcation, the blood vessels are less distinguishable because of their reduced diameter.

Despite the fact that the major blood vessels of the neck discussed previously are rarely distinguished from the rest of the soft tissues of the neck in CBCT images because of the limited soft tissue contrast (see Fig. 8), knowledge of and familiarity with the course of the blood vessel on the lateral neck is crucial to identify pathologic conditions inside or in the vicinity of the blood vessels, such as carotid artery atheromatosis, a pathologic condition in which calcified deposits (atheromas) accumulate on the internal wall of the blood vessel; this gradually reduces the flexibility and functionality of the blood vessel. Carotid artery atheromatosis demonstrates a fairly high incidence rate in older age groups and has been associated with an increased risk for stroke [3]. These calcifications most frequently occur within 10 to 15 mm of the bifurcation (above or below). Sometimes, they have a clear tubular appearance that makes them more readily identifiable than not. Other times, they look more like a cluster of calcifications in the region (Fig. 9).

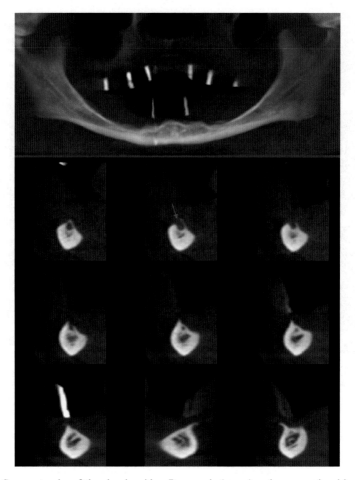

Fig. 6. Severe atrophy of the alveolar ridge. Panoramic (upper) and cross-sectional images of an edentulous patient who presented for preimplant assessment (see opaque markers on the crest of the alveolar ridge). The mandibular alveolar ridge demonstrates severe atrophy. The mental foramen now opens on the crest of the ridge (*red arrow*). Note the small well-defined lucent area just anterior to the mental foramen just inferior to the crest. This small channel hosts the continuation of the inferior alveolar nerve, which is known as the incisive branch of the inferior alveolar nerve. This continues towards the midline, past the mental foramen.

Other types of neck calcifications may include calcifications in the thyroid cartilage complex, stylohyoid ligament calcifications, sialoliths, and tonsilloliths (Figs. 10 and 11). Some may resemble carotid artery calcifications; however, the appearance and location should assist in determining the origin of the calcification most of the time.

Apart from the visualization of the corresponding cervical vertebrae (depending on the level of the axial sections) and the mandibular bone, axial images of the floor of the mouth reveal minimal information about the soft tissue structures in the region (Fig. 12).

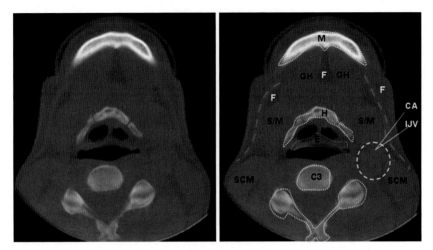

Fig. 7. (*Left*) Axial CBCT image at the level of the hyoid and C3 vertebra. (*Right*) Same axial image as the one on the left with some identifiable neck anatomic structures outlined (despite the fact that the soft tissue contrast of CBCT is not optimal for the diagnosis of soft tissue pathologic conditions, some of the neck anatomic landmarks are visualized). H, hyoid bone; M, inferior border of the anterior mandible. Note the almost modular appearance of the hyoid bone that can imitate a fracture. C3, axial section of the third cervical vertebra; E, epiglottis; F, fatty tissue; GH, geniohyoid muscle; SCM, sternocleidomastoid muscle; S/M, submandibular salivary glands. Because of the fact that they are mainly occupied by fat, the neck spaces appear of a lower density in comparison to the neighboring musculature. CA, carotid arteries, IJV, internal jugular vein. Please note that this is the approximate location of the major blood vessels of the neck; their precise location cannot be clearly seen without the use of intravenous administration of contrast media. Knowledge of the topographic location of the major neck anatomic structures can assist the diagnostician to determine the origin of the various pathologic entities that may develop on the neck.

Sagittal images of the neck are best for the assessment of the cervical spine and the airway (Fig. 13). The cervical spine is only partially visualized in a CBCT scan (C1–C4). The normal (healthy) appearance of the vertebral bodies includes a fairly square body, a thin cortical outline, a cancellous component of homogeneous density, and a fairly symmetric spacing between the vertebrae visible in the scan. Pathologic findings associated with the cervical spine and other irregularities are not uncommon. Often, these are incidental findings in scans that were prescribed for different reasons (see Fig. 13B, C).

The airway is identified as an irregularly shaped, elongated, low-density (dark) area anterior to the cervical part of the vertebral column. The position of the epiglottis, the laryngeal opening below the epiglottis, and the position of the tongue may have an effect on the diameter of the airway in several locations. CBCT images are useful in the evaluation of the airway and the factors that may cause restrictions in the airflow in sleep apnea cases (Fig. 14).

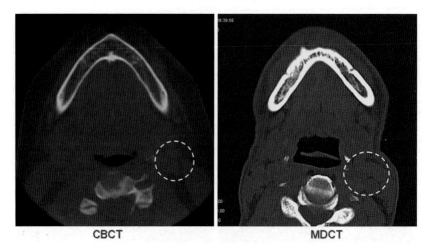

Fig. 8. Soft tissue contrast between CBCT and multidetector CT (MDCT). CBCT axial image at the level of C3 (*left*) and MDCT (*right*). Note the higher soft tissue contrast for MDCT images and the sharper depiction of structures like muscles and blood vessels, for example. The dotted ring outlines the region where the major blood vessels of the neck most frequently appear. The three round well-defined soft tissue structures seen in the marked area on the MDCT image medial to the SCM muscle may represent the carotid arteries and the internal jugular vein. On the contrary, the same region seems to be rather unclear in the CBCT axial image.

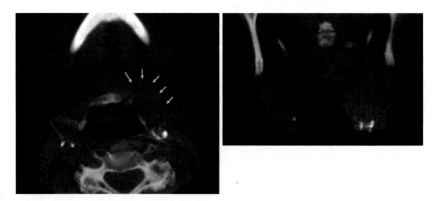

Fig. 9. Axial and coronal images of the neck. Bilateral circular calcifications are noted at the level of C3 and C4, toward the posterolateral wall of the airway, just medial to the anterior border of the SCM (*red arrows*). These are carotid artery calcifications attributable to atheromatosis. Note that the appearance of the left (L) calcification in the coronal image resembles the lumen of a vessel. Also, note the marked neck asymmetry between the right and left sides of the neck. This is attributable to prior surgical removal of the right submandibular (SM) gland. The left SM gland is outlined by the blue arrows.

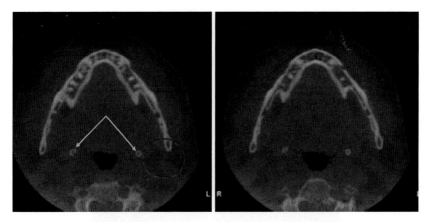

Fig. 10. Bilateral calcifications of the stylohyoid ligaments (*green arrows*). Note the close proximity to the location of the major blood vessels of the neck where carotid artery calcifications may occur (*round dotted region*). Also note the deep right and left submandibular gland depressions on the lingual aspect of the mandible (*Courtesy of* S. Thomas, DDS, MD, MS, Overland Park, KS).

The midfacial structures and the skull base are reviewed next in a series of axial sections (Figs. 15–20). Apart from the apices of the maxillary teeth, the hard palate, and the floor of the maxillary sinuses, the superior foramina (anteriorly) and the greater and lesser palatine foramina are visualized at that level. The former are the entrance of the nasopalatine canal and are located on the floor of the nasal cavity (inferior meatus), and they host the nasopalatine nerve. The latter serve as the opening to the greater and lesser palatine nerves and vessels that run the hard palate from posterior to anterior just superior to the palatal roots of the maxillary molars in the soft tissue in a palatal mucosa (see Fig. 15). Their identification during palatal

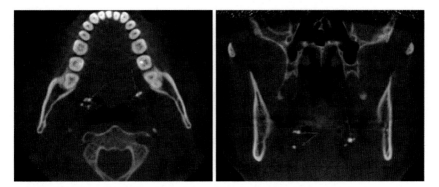

Fig. 11. Bilateral calcifications (*arrows*) at the level of the floor of the mouth (axial and coronal images). Note the superficial location of the calcifications in relation to the airway. These were tonsillar calcifications or tonsilloliths. These are frequently associated with recurrent inflammation of the tonsils.

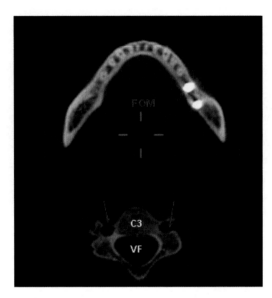

Fig. 12. Axial cut of the mandible toward the lower half of the mandibular body. At that level, the C3 vertebra is depicted. VF, vertebral foramen. The red arrows mark the right and left transverse foramen (or foramen transversarium). Contiguous transverse foramina form a canal that hosts the vertebral artery during its ascending course toward the endocranium. FOM, floor of the mouth. Note that because of inadequate soft tissue contrast, it is impossible to distinguish different soft tissue structures in the mouth.

surgery and palatal flap elevation is important. Similar to several other important anatomic structures, they cannot always be visualized in CBCT scans.

The nasopharyngeal aspect of the airway dominates the center of the axial cuts of the midface. Its shape and size varies and may be affected by neighboring anatomic structures in the vicinity. A deep depression on the lateral walls of the nasopharynx bilaterally is the Eustachian tube, the tube that communicates and balances the air pressure between the inner ear and external ear (see Fig. 15). Just posterior to the Eustachian tube, separated only by a soft tissue projection (torus tubarius), lies the pharyngeal recess or fossa of Rosenmüller. The fossa of Rosenmüller has been associated with pathologic entities. This region is almost always going to appear in the maxillary CBCT scans, and it is imperative that it be included in an evaluation. Further dorsally, an ovoid or ellipsoid structure is visualized toward the anterior aspect of the foramen magnum; this is the odontoid process of the axis (see Fig. 2, axial image).

Axial cuts made more cephalad reveal the right and left maxillary sinuses (see Fig. 16). Almost pyramidal in shape, with the base of the pyramid being the medial wall or the wall that is shared with the nasal cavity and the other two sides, are the anterior wall and the posterior wall. As mentioned

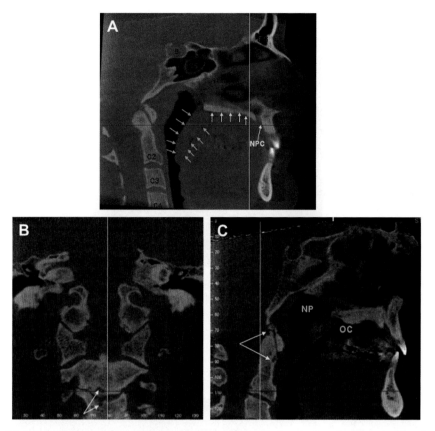

Fig. 13. (*A*) Midsagittal cut of the face and neck. Sagittal sections are best for the evaluation of the visible portion of the cervical spine and the airway. C2, second cervical vertebra-axis; C3, third cervical vertebra-axis; C4, fourth cervical vertebra-axis; FS, frontal sinus; NPC, nasopalatine canal; S, sella turcica; SS, sphenoid sinus. The yellow arrows mark the hard palate, and the green arrows mark the soft palate. The elongated, slightly curved, low-density area anterior to the cervical spine is the airway. Coronal (*B*) and sagittal (*C*) images of the same case demonstrate clear evidence of degenerative joint disease in the visible part of the cervical spine. The yellow arrows show erosive lesions or small subchondral cysts in the C2 and C3 vertebral bodies. Other signs of degenerative joint disease (arthritis) include loss of intervertebral space, osteophyte formation, and sclerosis, for example. In the sagittal image (*C*), the soft palate (SP) separates the upper airway into two distinct parts: the nasopharynx (NP) and the oral cavity (OC).

previously, all the air cavities are demonstrated as absolute black because of the fact that air is depicted as a low-density structure in CT. The presence of any other appearance other than black may represent a pathologic finding in the air cavity. As far as the nasal cavity is concerned, the structures being sectioned are elongated structures running the nasal cavity from anterior to posterior; these are the inferior nasal conchae and their soft tissue outline

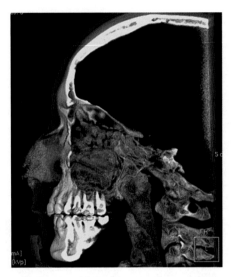

Fig. 14. A thick sagittal cut visualized in three dimensions to assess the airway shown in blue. Several software programs (mostly third party) offer specific utilities that simplify airway evaluation in addition to measurements and volume analysis, for example.

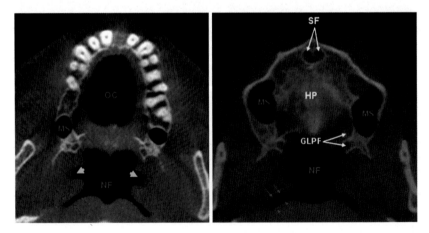

Fig. 15. (*Left*) Axial section at the level of the roots of the maxillary teeth. (*Right*) Axial section slightly superior to the other one, at the level of the floor of the maxillary sinus. GLPF, greater and lesser palatine foramina; HP, hard palate; MS, maxillary sinus; OC, oral cavity; SF, superior foramina, the starting point of the nasopalatine canal. The green arrows show the pharyngeal opening of the Eustachian tube, which helps in equalizing the pressure between the two sides of the eardrum. The red arrows mark fossa Rosenmüller. The torus tubarius (TT), a soft tissue process on either side of the nasopharynx separating the Eustachian tube, forms the fossa Rosenmüller.

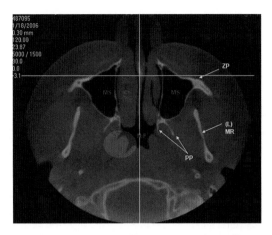

Fig. 16. Axial section at the level of the maxillary sinuses and mandibular rami demonstrates major structures of the maxillary sinus, nasal cavity, and nasopharynx at the axial plane. INC, inferior nasal concha; MR, mandibular ramus; MS, maxillary sinus; N/F, nasopharynx; PP, lateral and medial pterygoid plates; ZP, zygomatic process of the maxilla. The red arrows mark the Eustachian tube, and the round shaded region marks the general site of fossa Rosenmüller and torus tubarius.

(see Figs. 16 and 17). The nasal structures and the paranasal sinus are best visualized in coronal images (discussed elsewhere in this article).

Axial cuts toward the superior third of the maxillary sinuses show additional important anatomic structures (see Figs. 17 and 18). The dense

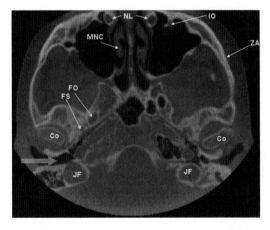

Fig. 17. Axial section at the level of the maxillary sinuses (superior third) demonstrates major structures of the maxillary sinuses, nasal cavity, and skull base at the axial plane. Co, mandibular condyle; FO, foramen ovale; FS, foramen spinosum; IO; infraorbital canal; JF, jugular foramen (or jugular fossa); Ma: mastoid air-cells; MNC, middle nasal concha; NL, nasolacrimal duct; SS, sphenoid sinus; ZA, zygomatic arch. The blue arrow indicates the external auditory canal.

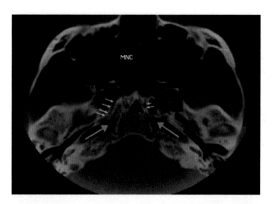

Fig. 18. Axial section at the level of the maxillary sinuses (superior third same as in Fig. 17, slightly higher) demonstrates additional anatomic details about the skull base. MNC, middle nasal concha; PPF, pterygopalatine fossa; SS, sphenoid sinus. The green arrows mark the walls of a thin channel known as the "Vidian canal" or pterygoid canal. The yellow arrows mark the course of the carotid canals, which appear to be converging toward the base of the sphenoid bone. The reader is reminded that the pterygopalatine fossa is a region of importance in the skull base. It is the passageway from the middle cranial fossa to the orbit, face, sinuses, and vice versa. Disease processes may be transferred from the middle cranial fossa to other sites (mentioned previously) through the pterygopalatine fossa. Similarly, disease originating extracranially may be transferred to the endocranium through the PPF.

arched-shaped structures seen on the lateral aspect of the face are the zygomatic arches. The anterior junction with the maxilla represents the zygomatomaxillary junction or suture in the anterior corner of the midface bilaterally.

The nasal septum is identified along the midline of the nasal cavity and is not always fully ossified. The middle nasal conchae are two of the osseous processes (six in total) that separate the nasal cavities in smaller chambers, the meati or turbinates. The two well-defined and well-corticated soft tissue content structures in the anterolateral wall of the nasal cavity bilaterally are the nasolacrimal ducts. The nasolacrimal ducts drain tears from the orbits to the inferior nasal turbinates.

Several important anatomic structures are identified posterior to the midface, in the skull base (see Figs. 17–19). These are the mandibular condyles, external auditory canals, and mastoid processes (partially visualized) bilaterally and the sphenoid sinus almost in the center of the axial image. Anteromedial to the mandibular condyles lay two important foramina: the foramen ovale (larger one) and the foramen spinosum (smaller one). The former hosts the third division of the trigeminal nerve (V3) and the mandibular nerve, and the latter hosts the middle meningeal artery.

At the same level, simply by slightly changing the reformatting angle to make our sections more parallel to the skull base, additional important anatomic structures appear. One of the most important anatomic regions

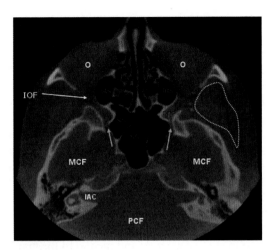

Fig. 19. Axial image of the head at level of the orbits (inferior third). The section depicts the roof of the maxillary sinuses bilaterally (MS) and the ethmoid sinuses (ES) just medial to the maxillary sinuses. Please note the fine and delicate air cells that form the ethmoid sinuses; this fine and complicated architecture has given the name of ethmoid labyrinth to the ethmoid air cells. The circular depressions toward the posterolateral walls of the sphenoid sinuses (SS), which can be seen in its magnitude in this image, represent the continuation of the carotid canals (CC) as they are entering the cavernous sinus of the lateral border of the base of the sphenoid bone. Note the septations present in the sphenoid sinus seen in this image. The section clearly illustrates the relation between the pterygopalatine fossa (PPF), the inferior orbital fissure (IOF), and the temporal fossa (*yellow dotted area*). Finally, the green arrows mark the course of the right and left foramen rotundum. IAC, internal auditory canal; MCF, middle cranial fossa; PCF, posterior cranial fossa.

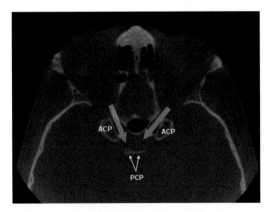

Fig. 20. Axial section of the head at the level of the orbits (superior half). The posterior opening of the orbits is divided to the superior orbital fissure (SOF) and the optic canal (*large yellow arrows*). The orientation of the optic canals is toward the sella turicica; this is the location of the optic chiasma. ACP, anterior clinoid processes; PCP, posterior clinoid processes.

of the skull base is the pterygopalatine fossa (PPF), which is identified in contact with the posterior wall of the right and left maxillary sinuses. The pterygopalatine fossa represents a major crossroad in the skull base. Two large osseous channels open in the PPF: the Vidian canal (or pterygoid canal), which hosts fibers of the petrosal nerves, and the foramen rotundum, which carries the maxillary nerve (V2). With the PPF as a passageway, the middle cranial fossa communicates with the orbits (through the inferior orbital fissure) and with the paranasal sinuses through the sphenopalatine foramen, the infratemporal fossa, and the nasal cavity. Through this crossroad, inflammation from the orbits, nasal cavity, sinuses, and oral cavity can be transferred into the middle cranial fossa and vice versa. The identification of the pterygopalatine fossa and assessment of the integrity of its margins are absolutely necessary if this structure is demonstrated in the CBCT scan [4,5].

Just posterior to the foramen ovale and medial to the mandibular condyle lays the carotid canal on either side of the skull base. The two canals converge toward the base of the sphenoid, where they pass close to the cavernous sinus before they ascend.

At the same level, almost in contact with the posterior border of the external auditory canals and medial to the mastoid air cells, the jugular foramina are visualized. Also known as jugular fossae (because of their large size), they are well defined, wide, corticated canals that serve as the passage points for the ninth, tenth, and eleventh cranial nerves and the jugular vein, among others. Variation in their shape and size in addition to asymmetry is not uncommon.

More cephalad sections (see Fig. 19) show the orbits, the ethmoid sinuses, and the sphenoid sinuses. The posterior opening of the orbits at that level is the inferior orbital fissure, which communicates with the pterygopalatine fossa as mentioned previously.

The ethmoid sinuses are made up of numerous, small, thin-walled air cells separated by the vomer bone (nasal septum), in the midline. Their complicated anatomy gave them the characterization of the ethmoid labyrinth.

The sphenoid sinus is located just posterior to the ethmoid sinuses. These are air cavities that are irregular in shape and size, located just below the base of the sphenoid bone. Anatomic variation and septations are often the rule rather than the exception.

As with all the air cavities that the author has defined and discussed so far, their healthy (normal) appearance is dark or black. When anything other than a dark appearance is noted, it may represent a pathologic entity in the region. The sinuses are evaluated and reviewed in more detail in the coronal images to visualize their relation to the nasal cavity and to each other better in addition to their draining.

The most superior axial sections reveal the upper half of the orbits, the temporal fossa, and parts of the middle and posterior cranial fossae. The concavities seen toward the posterolateral orbital walls are the temporal fossae; they are anatomic depressions into the temporal bone and serve as the attachment point for the temporalis muscle (see Fig. 20).

At this level, the posterior opening of the orbits appears to be splitting into two distinct openings. The one medially, which appears to be converging toward the sella turcica and finally joining the contralateral one, is the optic canal. The optic canals host the optic nerves, which converge on the sella, forming the optic chiasma. The other opening is the superior orbital fissure. The linear structure along the midline demonstrating a transverse orientation, just posterior to the optic chiasma, is the posterior clinoid processes (see Fig. 20).

The author continues with the review of several anatomic structures in the coronal plane. It is strictly recommended so as to utilize fully the potential of multiplanar imaging to review and synthesize or reformat not only the anatomic structures of concern or the areas of interest in all three planes but to reformat images along custom-made planes or any plane that helps to differentiate the pathologic entity of interest and all the anatomic structures of interest.

Coronal sections are used for the evaluation of anatomic structures that have a posteroanterior orientation. The paranasal sinuses, structures of the nasal cavity, and certain structures in the skull base are going to be optimally imaged in this view. In this article, the author reviews the anatomic structures of interest starting from anterior to posterior (Figs. 21–26).

At the level of maxillary premolars, the coronal sections reveal the anterior aspect of the maxillary sinuses, a small portion of the frontal sinuses, and the orbits. A canal is identified toward the inferomedial wall of the orbit

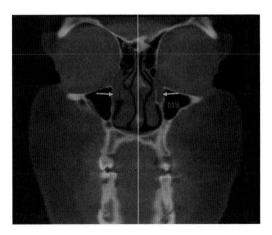

Fig. 21. Coronal section of the face approximately at the premolar level. The structures visualized at this level are the orbits (O), frontal sinuses (FS), oral cavity (OC), anterior walls of the right and left maxillary sinuses, and nasolacrimal ducts, marked by the green arrows.

ANGELOPOULOS

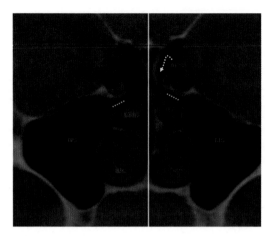

Fig. 22. Coronal section of the face approximately at the level of maxillary sinuses and nasal cavity (maxillary molar level). These images are optimal for the evaluation of the integrity of the floor and walls of the sinuses and nasal cavities. The draining site of the maxillary sinuses (osteomeatal complex) and ethmoid sinuses can be best evaluated in these sections (in this image, the draining channel is marked with a *green dotted line*). As you can see, the maxillary sinuses drain into the middle nasal turbinate (meatus). It is imperative that this structure is identified and assessed before possible sinus grafting procedures. The anterior ethmoid air cells (AES) drain close to those of the maxillary sinuses (*see curved yellow arrow*) in the middle nasal turbinate as well. INC, inferior nasal concha; MNC, middle nasal concha; MS, maxillary sinus.

(see Fig. 21); this is the nasolacrimal canal that originates on the floor of the orbit and drains into the inferior nasal turbinate.

The nasal anatomy and the anatomy of the maxillary sinuses can be reviewed best at the level of the maxillary molars. The nasal cavity is

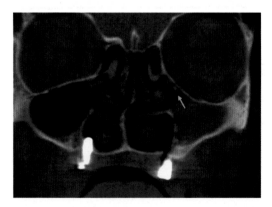

Fig. 23. Coronal section through the maxillary sinuses shows the presence of inflammatory tissue in the left maxillary sinus and thickening of the mucosal lining of the floor and walls of the right maxillary sinus. Note the blocked draining channel (ostium) marked by the green arrow.

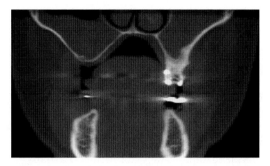

Fig. 24. Coronal section through the sinuses shows extensive inflammation (collection of soft tissue in density content in the sinus cavities) of the right and left maxillary sinuses. Also, note the severe pneumatization of the right sinus; it appears that the floor of the sinus and the crest of the alveolar ridge coincide.

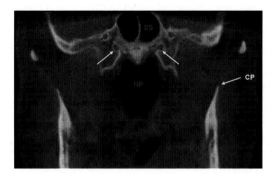

Fig. 25. Coronal section through the sphenoid sinus. CP, coronoid process of the mandible; NP, nasopharynx; SS, sphenoid sinus. The yellow arrows show the Vidian canal (pterygoid canal), and the red arrows show the foramen rotundum.

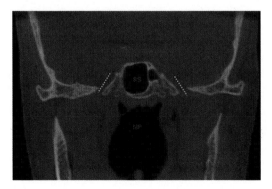

Fig. 26. Coronal section through the sphenoid sinus (just posterior to section in Fig. 25). SS, sphenoid sinus; NP, nasopharynx. The dotted green lines mark the course of the foramen ovale bilaterally.

separated into three distinct chambers (meati or turbinates) on either side of three osseous processes, the nasal conchae (inferior, middle, and superior). Only the inferior concha is an independent facial bone; the rest are parts of the ethmoid bone. The position of the nasal septum may contribute to the asymmetry between the right and left sides (see Fig. 22).

Coronal views toward the anterior third of the orbits will reveal the paper-thin plate of the ethmoid or lamina papyracea. At this level, the draining sites of the maxillary sinuses are likely to be visualized. In fact, they are narrow passageways toward the superomedial wall of the maxillary sinuses leading into the middle nasal turbinate; they are formed partially from the ethmoid bone (superior) and a thin pointy osseous process on the lateral wall of the nasal cavity known as the uncinate process. The site, as a whole, is known as the osteomeatal complex (see Fig. 22). Asymmetry between the right and left sides and variation from individual to individual are not uncommon. Identification of the draining sites and assessment of their integrity are important in patients who undergo sinus grafting procedures. Blockage of the draining site may prevent the aeration of the sinus cavity and result in accumulation of inflammatory products into the sinus (see Figs. 23 and 24). The fine detailed and delicate anatomy of the ethmoid sinuses may be grossly altered if prior sinus surgery has occurred.

Coronal sections through the sphenoid sinuses reveal the sphenoid sinus anatomy and variants. Last, most of the anatomic structures discussed previously in the axial plane can be identified in the coronal sections as well (see Figs. 25 and 26).

It is strongly recommended that to take advantage of the CBCT images in full, the diagnostician should be able to understand and apply the concept of multiplanar reformatting to the highest degree. It is in the dentist's hands to reveal the information related to each diagnostic task. In other words, our diagnostic efficiency is based on our sound knowledge of anatomy and on our skills to retrieve relevant diagnostic information.

References

[1] Kalpidis CD, Setayesh RM. Hemorrhaging associated with endosseous implant placement in the anterior mandible: a review of the literature. J Periodontol 2004;75(5):631–45.
[2] Tepper G, Hofschneider UB, Gahleitner A, et al. Computed tomographic diagnosis and localization of bone canals in the mandibular interforaminal region for prevention of bleeding complications during implant surgery. Int J Oral Maxillofac Implants 2001;16(1):68–72.
[3] Mupparapu M, Kim IH. Calcified carotid artery atheroma and stroke: a systematic review. J Am Dent Assoc 2007;138(4):483–92.
[4] Som PM, Curtin HD. Head and neck imaging. 3rd edition. St Louis (MO): Mosby; 1996.
[5] Harnsberger HR, Wiggins RH, Hudgins PA, et al. Diagnostic imaging head and neck. Manitoba (Canada): Canada Elsevier; 2005.

THE DENTAL CLINICS
OF NORTH AMERICA

Dent Clin N Am 52 (2008) 753–759

Application of Cone-beam CT in the Office Setting

Steven L. Thomas, DDS, MS

Thomas Oral Surgery, PC, 12800 Metcalf Avenue, Suite 2, Overland Park, KS 66213, USA

Rarely in the course of a person's career does a technique or technology come along that completely transforms the way they practice. In my case, two such events have happened, the most recent of which was the in-office availability of CT. As an oral and maxillofacial surgery resident and throughout my career, I have worked with three-dimensional imaging in the hospital setting, but the inconvenience for office-based patients and the cost prohibited its use in all but the most complicated cases. Even with high-quality digital panoramic and intraoral imaging, the third dimension of dental imaging was an educated guess based on experience, technique, and "rules" that I often found to give inconsistent results. Hospital and imaging center CT scans also had significant limitations because of the inability to manipulate the data. Multiplanar reconstruction was limited to axial, coronal, and sagittal views, and no customization was offered.

The advent of three-dimensional surgical planning software for implant placement, in my opinion, opened the door for the imaging opportunities that we now have available as office-based practitioners. Even though the software required the use of a traditional fan beam CT image file and multiple conversions, it put the data in the hands of the doctor, enabling him or her to make and change treatment decisions based on information that was specific to a region of interest. Further mining of the data allowed the creation of seemingly endless possibilities for diagnosis.

As office-based procedures have become more sophisticated and expectations have risen for highly successful outcomes, immediate and accurate information has become essential for treating our patients. Several cone beam acquisition machines are now on the market and even more software products to use the data. This time is an exciting one in dentistry, when we can reach beyond the limitations of our senses and the two-dimensional

E-mail address: thomas@thomasoralsurgery.com

world of the last century in dental radiology to see what's really happening in the mouth and its associated hard tissues.

Determining if cone-beam CT is right for your practice

Several factors need to be taken into consideration before purchasing a cone-beam CT (CBCT) device for your practice. Like any other large capital acquisition, it needs to benefit your patients and be affordable, either by generating income or by providing such significant information that it becomes essential to patient care. Although specialty practices lend themselves best as candidates for using the information in a CBCT, general practices can also benefit greatly, especially if they perform expanded function procedures.

Although the technology has not yet been perfected for accurate caries detection using the cone beam scanner, the three-dimensional scanning of all the roots of a tooth during endodontic treatment to detect perforation or aberrant canals is useful. That application alone can prevent the loss of countless numbers of teeth each year.

The time-honored method for monitoring periodontal bone loss has been through the use of a periodontal probe and bitewing radiographs. Although this method is inexpensive, it is technique-sensitive and does not allow full visualization of the area. In addition to added visualization with CBCT images, most software includes tools for evaluating and monitoring bone density, which may help assess the effectiveness of treatment, predict the results of treatment, or identify areas of future concern.

To paraphrase the most well-known line in real estate, what are the three most important things in dental implant treatment? Location, location, and location. Anyone involved in the placement and restoration of dental implants knows this to be true. The application of CBCT has changed this area more than any other in dentistry. From three-dimensional planning to CT-directed placement to take advantage of available bone and avoid anatomic structures, the science of implantology has been revolutionized by three-dimensional imaging. Not only has it added safety and accuracy; it has minimized or eliminated the need for supportive procedures like bone and tissue grafts in many situations. Computer-generated surgical guides can be fabricated from the CBCT data to eliminate the work and possible inaccuracy of taking impressions and making traditional guide stents.

In the areas of oral surgery and oral pathology, the data from the CBCT can have a profound impact on decision making. The location and root configuration of impacted and erupted teeth can be seen with exceptional clarity. The proximity to adjacent structures can be seen and measured with digital accuracy. The extension of periapical lesions, areas of bone destruction, and involvement of the maxillary sinus are all clearly defined. Even those "spots" seen on traditional radiography can be pinpointed and diagnosed, eliminating the question of artifact and allowing the dentist to give patients definitive diagnoses.

If your practice does not incorporate enough of these situations to justify acquiring your own CBCT scanner, consideration can be given to sharing the equipment and software with an affiliated practice. Because the information gleaned from the hardware is digital, it can easily be transferred around the corner or around the world. The best arrangements, however, are when the equipment is located in the same building or within walking distance of your practice. Otherwise, you lose one of the important considerations of CBCT for your patients, and that is convenience.

Facility evaluation

An important factor in deciding to implement CBCT in your practice is whether your current office location will accommodate the hardware and software. The earliest office-based CT scanners had complex mechanical requirements and needed significant amounts of space. Modern scanners can fit in the space of a standard panoramic radiograph machine. A dedicated electric circuit is required, but no special heating, ventilation, or air conditioning is routinely needed. Laws vary from state to state regarding radiation safety, but the new machines emit less radiation than older conventional radiograph machines and scan times of less than 10 seconds will soon be routine, lowering the radiation even more. Radiation monitoring is suggested, but our experience has been that the monthly exposure is negligible.

Most CBCT scanners come with the necessary hardware and software to operate the capture station, but making the data available to other computers on your network will be your responsibility. It may not be necessary in small office situations but it is likely that you will want the ability to access the data from multiple locations, so a reliable, high-speed network should be in place in your office. If you intend to transmit images to other offices, a high-speed Internet connection will also be necessary. Currently, the size of the files and the compression available will not allow the whole file to be sent electronically, at least in a practical sense, so printing reports as portable document files (.pdf) and sending them as attachments to e-mails has been a useful tool. Data can also be placed on a CD or DVD for delivery. Many systems include the software to read and manipulate the data as a free service and the systems will copy to the disk when the data are burned.

Acquiring the skills to interpret cone-beam CT

Specialists who train in hospital-based residencies are usually exposed to various advanced techniques in radiology, especially CT. Oral and maxillofacial radiology residencies spend a considerable amount of time training residents in the use of fan beam and CBCT. But what about the general practitioner who wants to incorporate CBCT into his/her practice? This problem is probably the biggest challenge and the biggest opportunity for the dental community and for the industries that provide the hardware and software. As dentists, we are technically oriented, and learning to operate the equipment requires a short amount of training and practice. Traditional dental radiographs (panoramic, cephalometric, periapical, and occlusal images) can be made from the data and interpreting these data is no different from interpreting those obtained by film techniques. The difference is all of the additional data that are acquired and available. Mini-residencies and short courses are available for several products and techniques and these are becoming more widely available for CBCT. If you are considering the addition of CBCT, you need to be prepared for this issue, because self training can only provide a limited amount of knowledge. Dental schools are beginning to discuss interpretation of CBCT in their curriculum but only to a limited degree. The answer may lie in the use of a specialty reading service.

To consult or not to consult

Because the data are digital, they can be accessed and interpreted with ease by an individual at a distant site. Many oral and maxillofacial radiologists offer analysis and interpretation of CBCT data at a reasonable cost, either on a case-by-case basis or by providing analysis of all your patients on a regular basis. This analysis is usually done by allowing the radiologist remote access to your image acquisition computer by using a high-speed data transmission line. The analysis can be in-depth if a specific concern exists or can be a cursory review to ensure that pathology does not go unrecognized. These reports are then e-mailed back to the dentist for review and inclusion in the patient's record. The professional fee for this service varies with the volume and type of analysis but should be considered when determining how much to charge for the scan.

The question of liability is one that frequently comes up in the discussion of CBCT. What happens if you fail to diagnose a condition that was clearly visible on the scan? To date, I am not aware of any liability case where failure to diagnose has been the basis for a claim. Nonetheless, it remains a real concern. If the dentist is only able to interpret traditional dental radiographs, then it makes sense to only reconstruct those images and to only charge the patient for those images. Findings outside of the oral cavity and jaws may be visible, as they are on panoramic or cephalometric films, but no clear-cut answer exists as to whether the dentist has an obligation to diagnose them. Soft tissue lesions, the ones most likely to be dangerous and the hardest to interpret, are not readily viewed using CBCT so it is unlikely that a tumor in the brain, for instance, would be "missed" by the dentist reading the scan. That being said, our responsibility to our patients is to provide them the best care we can. If you are going to incorporate CBCT into your practice you should make the effort to learn how to interpret those data and have a radiologist available to consult when needed.

Transition to the third dimension: leaving the past behind?

Several issues need to be considered when making the decision to expand into three-dimensional radiography and retaining your traditional film or digital equipment depends on your scope of practice. If you have a highly subspecialized practice like implantology, you may find that CBCT alone can meet all your needs. CBCT does have limitations at this time that will require most practices to retain some, if not all, of their current equipment. Caries detection is not yet something that can be consistently done with CBCT. Pediatric patients, uncooperative patients, and those who have neuromuscular disorders often cannot remain quiet for the time necessary to acquire the data. Any movement during the scan will render it useless. Claustrophobic patients and those who are tall or wide may have trouble with positioning. Although the radiation dose is small considering the amount of data that is acquired, patients requiring serial examinations may not need a full scan and would be better served with traditional studies for follow-up. At a minimum, the ability to take intraoral radiographs should be maintained until it is determined that it is no longer necessary.

Speaking in code

If your practice files claims with insurance companies, you will need to know the current dental terminology and current procedural terminology codes that apply to CBCT to gain reimbursement for your patients. Box 1 provides much of that information, but the diagnosis code must be specific to each patient's situation. It should be borne in mind that the existence of a code for the service provided does not mean it is a covered benefit and that some medical insurance companies have limitations on who can bill for certain services.

Health Insurance Portability and Accountability Act and security

We are all familiar with the Health Insurance Portability and Accountability Act (HIPAA) and the need for securing our patient's protected health care information. Because may offices are now paperless or partially paperless, the protection of the digital information from the CBCT will not require any major change in policy. Because the data will contain some personal information about the subject, safeguards do need to be taken when transmitting these data for analysis or additional opinions from consultants. If someone who is not affiliated with your practice, such as an oral and maxillofacial radiologist, is evaluating the data, it is recommended that an agreement be in place that includes a statement of confidentiality. This agreement is not necessary when working with another dentist or physician in the treatment of a patient, but a disclaimer about confidentiality should be present when the images are sent electronically. Also, if the images are

---

Box 1. Diagnosis and procedure codes

Procedures
  CDT 00363: CBCT
  CPT 70486: CT (maxillofacial without contrast)
Common ICD9 codes
  307.81: Headache, tension
  351.9: Disorder, facial nerve
  520.6: Disturbance, tooth eruption
  523.4: Periodontitis, chronic
  524.9: Anomaly, dentofacial
  525.2: Atrophy, edentulous alveolar ridge
  526.0: Cysts, development odontogenic
  526.4: Inflammation, jaw
  714.0: Arthritis, rheumatoid
  716.18: Arthritis, traumatic
  733.00: Osteoporosis
  784.2: Swelling in head/neck
  802.: Fracture
  830.0: Dislocation, closed jaw
  830.1: Dislocation, open jaw
  848.1: Sprain/strain, jaw

---

to be used during professional presentations, any identifying information should be removed.

Data storage

Never believe someone who tells you your hard drive has all the capacity you will ever need! The need for speed and storage will always exceed capacity, especially with the use of highly specialized programs. The data compression with most CBCT equipment has improved but the records must be maintained and each image from the i-CAT (Imaging Sciences) is approximately 45 MB. If you have a busy practice, you will quickly exceed the storage space that comes with the acquisition computer. Fortunately, data storage prices have fallen recently and hard drives in the 500 gigabyte to 1 terabyte range are readily affordable. It is important to plan ahead because the machines will slow down significantly when data storage space is limited.

Data backup is also a concern. Most users have found it impractical to burn a CD of each patient's data to place in a chart. HIPAA regulations, and common sense, indicate that an off-site backup is necessary because for most of us, the volume of data is too large to use an online backup service. Tape backups can be performed and taken off site but they are slow and often require a significant number of tapes. Services are available that keep your original data off site in a secure location and allow you to run your office remotely, which is a great way to protect your information, but the cost is often prohibitive and the speed of data transmission may make it impractical.

In my office, I have found that the use of 500-gigabyte portable hard drives provides the fastest and most practical backup. Two drives are rotated daily and one is always out of the office. They connect to the network and back up all the data overnight so they do not interfere with daily activities. These hard drives are light and compact and recovery, should it be necessary, is quick.

Marketing: internal and external

Marketing is one of those words that often make us uncomfortable in a professional context, but in reality we do it every day, whether it is taking good care of the patients we have, handing out material at a health fair, or advertising in print or other media. Each of us must find our own comfort level. When it comes to CBCT, several possibilities exist. At a minimum, most practices will make it known through a newsletter or other form of communication to their current patients and colleagues that they have incorporated CBCT. If you are planning to expand the scope of your practice through the use of CBCT, you may wish to market further into the professional and lay community. Most CBCT suppliers can help by providing examples of press releases and can add you to their Web sites if they have sections to assist patients in trying to locate doctors who have CBCT capability. Your own Web site is a great way to make your patients and potential patients aware of the services you have to offer. Additionally, most radio and television stations have community service programming at no charge. These programs are constantly looking for interesting stories that can benefit their audience and the acquisition of cutting-edge technology by members of the community is a popular topic.

Looking back

The decision to incorporate CBCT into your practice is one that requires serious consideration and careful planning. I have used it in my practice since 2004 and feel it is an indispensable tool. In the early days of the technology, fewer sources of information existed and a community of users often shared ideas and prompted the advancement of the products. Office-based CBCT has advanced significantly since that time. It has often been described as the "gold standard" for imaging the oral and maxillofacial area and will no doubt become a part of the everyday life of most practices in the coming decades.

ELSEVIER
SAUNDERS

THE DENTAL
CLINICS
OF NORTH AMERICA

Dent Clin N Am 52 (2008) 761–775

Computer-Aided Dental Implant Planning

Leonard Spector, DDS

Spector + Krupp, DDS, PA, Oral and Maxillofacial Surgery,
1220 E. Joppa Road, Suite 314, Towson, MD 21286, USA

Advances in implant dentistry over the past 40 years have allowed for the predictable replacement of missing teeth [1–3]. It is now commonplace to treatment plan partially and fully edentulous areas in the mouth with implant-supported restorations. In the standard planning for a dental implant case, the doctor procures mounted dental models and designs a model-based surgical guide. Conventional dental radiographs and CT scans help the practitioner determine where the underlying bone relates to the final prosthesis [4]. But in most cases, to determine the anatomy of the alveolar ridge, the surgery requires a crestal incision with subperiosteal reflection of the gingiva, a method that can inadvertently displace the model-based surgical guide. Only in those cases that present with excess amounts of alveolar bone can the implant be placed in a flapless manner. Even with a model-based surgical guide, much depends on the skill of the operator in placing the implant in the preplanned position. The use of model-based guides to position dental implants becomes even more demanding in placing multiple implants, as in an edentulous arch with limited bone available.

In the past few years, technologic advances in interactive three-dimensional CT software have enabled the practitioner to treatment plan and place dental implants more predictably [5,6]. Computer-based planning is used to plan implant placement in partially edentulous (single tooth, multiple teeth) and, more often, fully edentulous cases involving a single arch or both arches. One surgical planning software, Procera Planning Software (Nobel Biocare, Yorba Linda, California), converts the patient's CT scan data into a three-dimensional model of the patient's facial bones and

---

The author holds no financial interest in Nobel Biocare or any other companies noted in this article.

E-mail address: lenspector@comcast.net

generates a three-dimensional representation of the proposed prosthesis in relation to the underlying alveolar ridge. The implants can be virtually placed in optimal sites, taking into account the patient's bone anatomy and the overlying position of the prosthesis. The computer-based plan is then used to create a customized surgical template that precisely guides the placement of the implants during surgery (NobelGuide). The dental laboratory uses the surgical template to fabricate the master cast and the provisional or final prosthesis.

The computer-based guided implant placement approach has numerous advantages. The presurgical planning and surgery are prosthetically driven and emphasize the team approach among the restorative dentist, surgeon, and dental laboratory. The surgeon can place the implants in their optimal and exact positions more accurately, predictably, and safely, as planned in the virtual software. Vital structures, such as adjacent tooth roots and the inferior alveolar nerve, can be avoided. The surgical template is so precise that the implants can be placed in minimal amounts of available bone, including those cases that would traditionally require bone grafting. In the severely atrophic maxilla, pterygomaxillary implants can be placed accurately with the use of the surgical template [7]. The minimally invasive guided surgery is performed without raising a flap, thereby minimizing postoperative pain and swelling and postoperative recovery time [8,9]. The chair time and number of appointments are also reduced, facilitating many patients' busy lifestyles. With the information contained within the surgical template, the dental laboratory can presurgically construct the master cast and the subsequent fabrication of a provisional restoration that can be inserted at the time of surgery (Teeth-in-an-Hour) or soon thereafter. Clinical studies support the long-term success of immediately loaded implants placed in a flapless manner and restored with a fixed complete restoration [10,11].

This article describes the process of computer-based guided implant surgery and the placement of an immediate provisional fixed prosthesis using Nobel Biocare's Procera planning software and the NobelGuide treatment approach, as performed in the author's office setting.

Presurgical evaluation and planning

The surgeon initially evaluates the patient with a thorough clinical and radiograph examination, including a preliminary cone-beam CT scan (also known as cone-beam volumetric tomography scan), digital photographs, and mounted dental models. The amount of available bone is assessed and nonrestorable teeth are identified. The nonrestorable teeth are removed and extraction sockets are bone grafted along with areas that have insufficient bone volume to place implants. The extraction sockets and bone grafts are allowed to consolidate completely. The patient must be able to open his/her mouth sufficiently to accommodate the additional 10-mm length of the burs used with the surgical template to prepare the implant sites.

The restorative dentist then fabricates dentures with the teeth in the ideal centric occlusion and in appropriate position for phonetics, aesthetics, and vertical dimension. The position of the teeth will be duplicated in the final fixed restoration, so the patient and practitioner must agree to the set-up. The prosthesis is made of acrylic and should not include a radiopaque liner. The denture should have exceptional soft tissue adaptation with an exact fit to the underlying mucosa. The flanges should be a minimum of 3-mm thick and overextended into the buccal and labial vestibules. In partially edentulous cases, once the ideal occlusion is established, an additional 3-mm thickness of acrylic is added to cover the occlusal surfaces of the existing teeth, and inspection windows are placed. The palate is also covered with acrylic to stabilize the denture further. In mandibular cases, the denture is extended to cover the retromolar area. All the features of the denture are reproduced in the surgical template.

The denture, or an exact duplicate, is then prepared as the radiographic guide. Ten to twelve fiducial markers are placed in a staggered pattern and at different levels to the occlusal plane on the buccal flanges and palatal and lingual surfaces. Each site is prepared with a #4 round bur to approximately 2-mm wide and 1.5-mm deep and filled with gutta percha (Coltene-Whaledent, Cuyahoga Falls, Ohio) (Fig. 1). A rigid vinyl polysiloxane bite registration, taken in centric occlusion, will be used to stabilize the radiographic guide against the opposing dentition during the CT scanning procedure.

Two cone-beam CT scans are made, with acquisition slices of 0.4 mm: the first, of the patient wearing the radiographic guide while occluding into the bite registration, and the second, of the radiographic guide alone, positioned in approximately the same orientation as in the first scan. These two Digital Imaging and Communication in Medicine (DICOM)-3 formatted files are

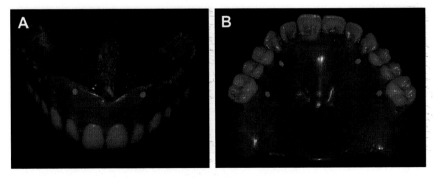

Fig. 1. (*A, B*) Ten to twelve gutta percha fiducial markers are placed in a staggered pattern, converting the patient's denture into the radiographic guide.

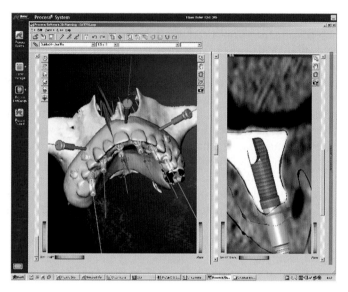

Fig. 2. The Procera planning software uses a three-dimensional computer-generated image of the maxilla and prosthesis (radiographic guide) to plan the placement of the implants. The two-dimensional screen on the right shows the cross-sectional re-slice of the alveolar bone and implant in area #8. (*Courtesy of* Nobel Biocare, Yorba Linda, CA; with permission.)

then imported into the Procera planning software and the data are converted into three-dimensional representations of the patient's alveolar bone and of the radiographic guide. The radiographic markers allow for the fusion of these two scans, thereby showing the relationship of the denture teeth to the underlying bone.

The virtual placement of the implants can now be performed. The Procera planning software uses a three-dimensional screen and a two-dimensional panel (Fig. 2). Both screens interrelate, so changes shown in

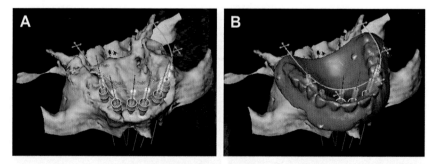

Fig. 3. The prosthesis has been hidden, to view the position of the implants in the maxilla (*A*), then displayed, to show the relationship of the implant abutments to the teeth (*B*). (*Courtesy of* Nobel Biocare, Yorba Linda, CA; with permission.)

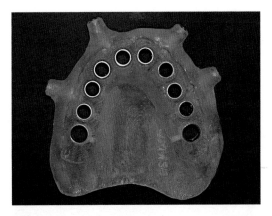

Fig. 4. A stereolithically processed maxillary surgical template from Nobel Biocare with 10 stainless steel drill guides and four lateral sleeves for the stabilization pins. The acrylic resin is light and moisture sensitive; to prevent warping, it should be stored in the protective UV bag that is delivered with the surgical template.

one screen are visualized in the other. The two-dimensional view allows for visualization of cross-sections of the alveolar bone along a slice curve in the three-dimensional screen. Using three-dimensional and cross-sectional views of the alveolar bone, along with an image of the overlying virtual prosthesis in exact relationship to the underlying bone, the implants can be virtually placed in the bone in relation to the position of the teeth in the final prosthesis. The three-dimensional image can be rotated in all spatial planes to assess the bony anatomy. The implant abutment and guide sleeve of the surgical template can be placed with each implant. The internal diameter of the guide sleeves corresponds precisely to the diameters of the drill guides and implants. Depending on which details need to be visualized, certain features

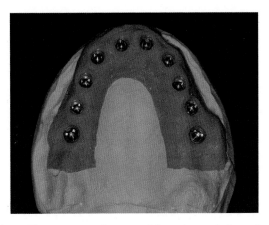

Fig. 5. The master cast is prepared from the surgical template.

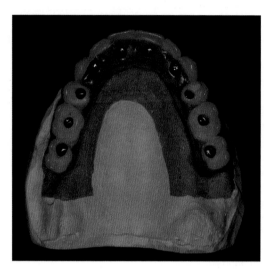

Fig. 6. A provisional fixed, all-acrylic, screw-retained prosthesis on the master cast.

of the virtual plan can be displayed or hidden (eg, the prosthesis, cross-sectional reslices, bone, or implant abutments) (Fig. 3). Additionally, horizontal stabilization pins (a minimum of one in partially edentulous cases and up to four in edentulous cases) are virtually placed through the labial denture flange to anchor the surgical template during surgery. After the restorative dentist and surgeon approve the virtual treatment plan, the three-dimensional computer planning files are digitally sent through the Internet to the Procera manufacturing facility (Nobel Biocare) for fabrication of the stereolithically constructed surgical template (Fig. 4). A map is

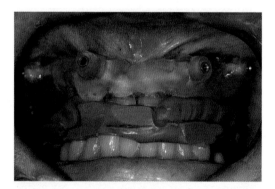

Fig. 7. The surgical template is positioned as the patient applies light pressure while occluding into the surgical index. Note the blanching of the underlying mucosa resulting from the exact fit of the surgical template.

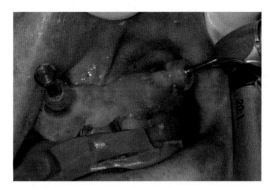

Fig. 8. The surgical template secured with stabilization pins.

printed from the planning software, depicting the size and location of each implant within the surgical template.

Approximately 2 weeks later, the surgical template is delivered to the office and a try-in is scheduled to confirm the accuracy of its fit. Thin and undersupported areas of the surgical template are reinforced with light-cured Triad gel (Dentsply International, York, Pennsylvania). In cases where an immediate provisional restoration is not planned, the patient can now be scheduled for surgery. For those cases in which an immediate provisional prosthesis will be inserted at the time of surgery or soon

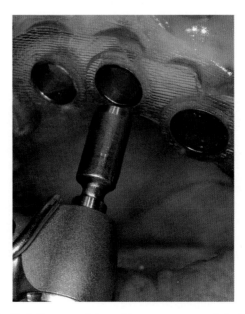

Fig. 9. A tissue punch is used to remove a core of gingiva.

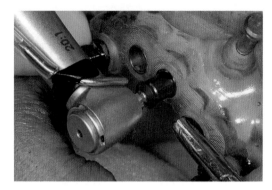

Fig. 10. Initial preparation is begun with the counterbore twist drill.

thereafter, the surgical template is sent to the dental laboratory, along with an opposing dental model, duplicate denture, and the interocclusal index used with the radiographic guide during the CT scan. The exactness of the surgical template allows for the presurgical construction of the master cast (Fig. 5) and the subsequent presurgical fabrication of a provisional restoration (Fig. 6) [12–14]. The dental laboratory uses the duplicate denture and interocclusal index to mount the master cast anatomically against the opposing dentition. A surgical index of rigid vinyl polysiloxane is prepared of the surgical template positioned on the articulated master cast occluding with the opposing dentition. The provisional restoration, surgical index, articulated models, and abutment components are delivered to the office and the patient is scheduled for surgery.

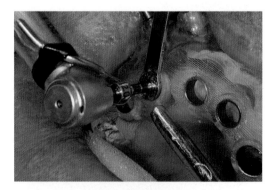

Fig. 11. The twist drill and corresponding twist-drill sleeve allow accurate preparation of the implant site. Each bur is 10-mm longer than a conventional bur to accommodate the distance (10 mm) between the top of the metal drill sleeve in the surgical template and the top of the implant.

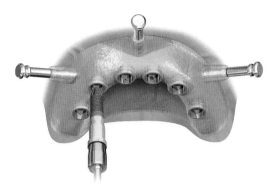

Fig. 12. The implant is connected to a guided implant mount and inserted into the prepared osteotomy. Care is taken not to overtighten the implant, which can result in the surgical template fracturing or becoming displaced. (*Courtesy of* Nobel Biocare, Yorba Linda, CA; with permission.)

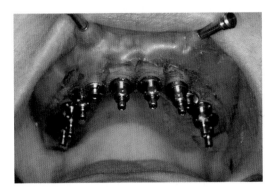

Fig. 13. Two template abutments are placed on the first two implants to stabilize the surgical template; the remaining implants are then placed.

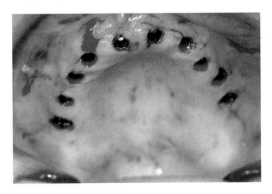

Fig. 14. The surgical template is removed and the implant sites are inspected.

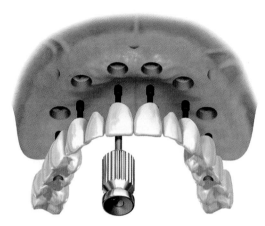

Fig. 15. The provisional restoration is connected to the implants with either screw-retained expanding guided abutments or multiunit abutments. (*Courtesy of* Nobel Biocare, Yorba Linda, CA; with permission.)

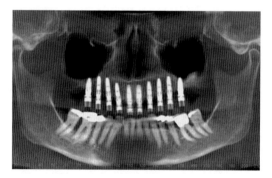

Fig. 16. Postoperative panoramic radiograph showing parallel alignment of 10 maxillary Nobel Speedy Replace implants placed with NobelGuide. Note the precise seating of the guided abutments on the implants.

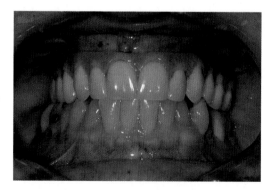

Fig. 17. Postoperative occlusion of the provisional restoration.

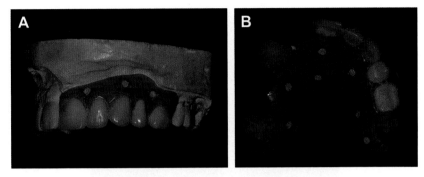

Fig. 18. In a partially edentulous case, additional acrylic is added to the radiographic guide to cover the occlusal aspect of some teeth (*A*) and the palate (*B*) to stabilize the surgical template.

Surgical procedure

Once the patient is prepared and draped and, if necessary, sedated, local anesthesia is injected, and the surgical template is placed and positioned with the surgical index. The patient is instructed to occlude into the index for 10 minutes to dissipate the local anesthesia, thereby ensuring that the surgical template is exactly seated on the underlying mucosa (Fig. 7). Then, with the patient biting firmly into the surgical index, a 1.5-mm twist drill is used to prepare the stabilization pin sites, the pins are placed (Fig. 8), and the surgical index is removed. A tissue punch (Fig. 9) is used to remove a core of gingiva from each guide sleeve and the initial implant preparation is begun with the counterbore starter drill (Fig. 10). Successive-sized twist drills with drill-stops are used with corresponding twist drill sleeves to prepare each implant site to the exact position and depth as determined in the virtual plan (Fig. 11). The preparation is undersized in diameter in soft bone, and in dense bone, a bone tap is used after the final width of the implant site is prepared. All burs are externally irrigated with copious amounts of cold saline, and the burs are used in a "pumping" fashion to allow the irrigant to flow to the apex of the preparation to prevent overheating of the bone. The implant is connected to a guided implant mount (Fig. 12) and inserted into the prepared osteotomy site with the torque wrench or implant drill. The implant is inserted to the depth at which the implant mount contacts the drill guide sleeve in the surgical template. Overtightening the implant can displace, and possibly fracture, the surgical template. In softer bone, overtightening can cause the implant threads to strip the preparation, and the implant will "spin," losing its initial stability in bone. In edentulous cases, after the initial two implants are placed, the guided implant mounts are removed and template abutments with expanding sidewalls that contact the inner aspect of the guide sleeves are placed on the initial two implants. These abutments further stabilize the surgical template while the additional

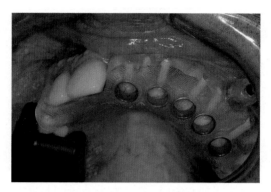

Fig. 19. NobelGuide surgical template for partially edentulous maxilla. Note the single lateral sleeve for the stabilization pin.

implant sites are prepared (Fig. 13). For a partially edentulous case, usually only one template abutment is needed.

Following the placement of the implants, the guided implant mounts, template abutments, and stabilization pins are removed and the surgical template is then removed. The implant sites are inspected and any residual overlying soft tissue is excised (Fig. 14). The provisional restoration is connected to the implants with either the screw-retained expanding guided abutments or multiunit abutments (Nobel Biocare, Loma Linda, California) (Fig. 15). Postoperative diagnostic images confirm the precise seating of the implant abutments on the implants (Fig. 16). Usually, minimal occlusal adjustments are needed. Fully edentulous cases are immediately loaded (Fig. 17). The screw access holes in the provisional restoration are then filled with a pledget of cotton and sealed with light cured Fermit (Ivoclar North America, Amherst, New York). Partially edentulous cases are either kept out of occlusion or placed with light occlusal contacts with delayed loading.

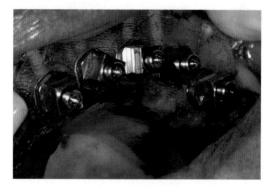

Fig. 20. Seating of five Nobel Speedy Groovy implants with guided implant mounts.

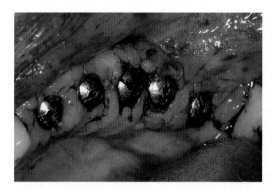

Fig. 21. Healing caps placed following removal of the surgical template.

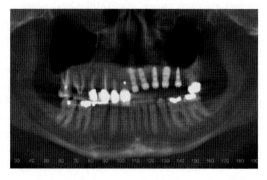

Fig. 22. Postoperative radiograph showing parallelism of the five guided implants.

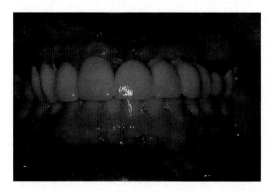

Fig. 23. Five individual porcelain-fused-to-metal crowns as final restorations.

In those cases where an immediate provisional restoration is not planned, bone-level impressions are taken and healing caps are placed (Figs. 18–23).

Postoperative instructions, including maintaining a soft diet for 6 weeks, rinsing with 0.12% chlorhexidine gluconate solution, using a water pick, and flossing techniques are reviewed with the patient before discharge. The patient, seen for a follow-up examination within the first week after surgery, typically has minimal postoperative pain and no swelling. The final fixed complete arch restoration, either a titanium-milled bar with acrylic teeth or a metal-ceramic restoration, is delivered 6 to 12 months later. In cases in which the final restoration is a partially edentulous prosthesis or clip-on denture, the prosthesis is seated following osseointegration of the implants.

Summary

Technologic advances in computed-based planning of implants has allowed the clinician to plan more accurately and place dental implants more precisely. With the Nobel Biocare Procera planning software, the virtual treatment plan is used to create a surgical template that guides the placement of the implants during surgery (NobelGuide). The minimally invasive surgery is performed without raising a flap, thereby minimizing surgery time, postoperative pain and swelling, and recovery time. The dental laboratory uses the information stored in the surgical template to fabricate presurgically a master cast and provisional restoration that can be placed immediately after surgery (Teeth-in-an-Hour). With the surgical template, the surgeon can place implants with accuracy, in areas of existing bone that, with conventional dental implant surgery, would require site preparation with bone grafting.

The use of computer-guided implant surgery has greatly enhanced the dental implant team's ability to plan, place, and restore implants accurately, with a level of precision that was unattainable a few years ago. It offers the patient an advanced level of care with reduced treatment time and a predictable final result.

References

[1] Branemark PI, Adell R, Breine U, et al. Intra-osseous anchorage of dental prostheses. I. Experimental studies. Scand J Plast Reconstr Surg 1969;3(2):81–100.

[2] Adell R, Lekholm U, Rockler B, et al. A 15-year study of osseointegrated implants in the treatment of the edentulous jaw. Int J Oral Surg 1981;10:387–416.

[3] Adell R, Eriksson B, Lekholm U, et al. Long-term follow-up study of osseointegrated implants in the treatment of totally edentulous jaws. Int J Oral Maxillofac Implants 1990; 5:347–59.

[4] Benson BW. Presurgical radiographic planning for dental implants. Oral Maxillofac Surg Clin North Am 2001;13:751–61.

[5] Parel SM, Triplett RG. Interactive imaging for implant planning, placement, and prosthesis construction. J Oral Maxillofac Surg 2004;9:41–7.

[6] Balshi SF, Wolfinger GJ, Balshi TJ. Surgical planning and prosthesis construction using computed tomography, CAD/CAM technology, and the Internet for immediate loading of dental implants. J Esthet Restor Dent 2006;18:312–23.

[7] Balshi SF, Wolfinger GJ, Balshi TJ. Surgical planning and prosthesis construction using computer technology and medical imaging for immediate loading of implants in the ptery-gomaxillary region. Int J Periodontics Restorative Dent 2006;26:239–47.

[8] Campelo LD, Camara JR. Flapless implant surgery: a 10-year clinical retrospective analysis. Int J Oral Maxillofac Implants 2002;17:271–6.

[9] Rocci A, Martignoni M, Gottow J. Immediate loading in the maxilla using flapless surgery, implants placed in predetermined positions, and prefabricated provisional restorations: a retrospective 3-year clinical study. Clin Implant Dent Relat Res 2003;5(Suppl 1):29–36.

[10] van Stenberghe D, Glauser R, Blomback U, et al. A computed tomographic scan-derived customized surgical template and fixed prosthesis for flapless surgery and immediate loading of implants in fully edentulous maxillae: a prospective multicenter study. Clin Implant Dent Relat Res 2005;7(Suppl 1):111–2.

[11] Kupeyan HK, Shaffner M, Armstrong J. Definitive CAD/CAM-guided prosthesis for imme-diate loading of bone-grafted maxilla: a case report. Clin Implant Dent Relat Res 2006;8(3): 161–7.

[12] Bedrossian E. Laboratory and prosthetic considerations in computer-guided surgery and immediate loading. J Oral Maxillofac Surg 2007;65(Suppl 1):47–52.

[13] Marchack CB. An immediately loaded CAD/CAM-guided definitive prosthesis: a clinical report. J Prosthet Dent 2005;93:8–12.

[14] Marchack CB. CAD/CAM-guided implant surgery and fabrication of an immediately loaded prosthesis for a partially edentulous patient. J Prosthet Dent 2007;97:389–94.

THE DENTAL
CLINICS
OF NORTH AMERICA

Dent Clin N Am 52 (2008) 777–808

Computer-aided Design/Computer-aided Manufacturing Applications Using CT and Cone Beam CT Scanning Technology

Scott D. Ganz, DMD[a,b,*]

[a]*Prosthodontics, Maxillofacial Prosthetics & Implant Dentistry,
158 Linwood Plaza, Suite 204, Fort Lee, NJ 07024, USA*
[b]*Department of Restorative Dentistry, University of Medicine and Dentistry
of New Jersey, Newark, NJ, USA*

Clinicians have been diagnosing, treatment planning, placing, and restoring modern dental implants using periapical and panoramic imaging films to assess bone anatomy for several decades. Two-dimensional film images have been found to have limitations because of inherent distortion factors, and the non-interactive nature of film itself provides little information regarding bone density, bone width, or spatial proximity of vital structures [1]. Digital radiography permits some interaction to enhance diagnostic interpretation but ultimately remains two dimensional (2-D). It was not until CT scan technology became available for dental applications that the three-dimensional (3-D) properties of the jawbones and vital structures became apparent. The advent of 3-D reconstruction using CT or cone beam CT (CBCT) empowers clinicians with tools to simulate implant placement, bone grafts, or orthognathic surgical procedures in a true and accurate virtual environment [2–4]. There are three basic views that a CT scan will provide: (1) panoramic, (2) axial, and (3) cross-sectional. The fourth view contains the 3-D reconstruction, and may differ in quality depending on the scanning machine and the software that is used to manage the CT data.

The original films that were the products of these scans provided clinicians with ample information, but no interactive ability, and therefore limited the diagnostic capabilities or the potential for collaboration with other

* Prosthodontics, Maxillofacial Prosthetics & Implant Dentistry, 158 Linwood Plaza, Suite 204, Fort Lee, NJ 07024.
E-mail address: sdgimplant@aol.com

technologies such as CAD/CAM (computer-aided design/computer-aided manufacturing). However, when innovative software applications permitted CT scan data to be viewed and manipulated on a desktop or laptop computer, a new world of anatomic realization was introduced. True, undistorted representations of the mandible or maxilla, combined with an array of tools for accurate treatment planning of realistic dental implants, abutments, and restorations are now possible. Manufacturer-specific CAD files have now been incorporated into libraries of data that can be manipulated within the framework of the virtual world of 3-D CT scan imaging. It is the combined enhanced capability of innovative software applications that allow clinicians to interpret and maneuver through various 3-D images that has far-reaching implications that will be explored in this article through the use of interactive treatment planning software in collaboration with computer-aided design and manufacturing.

Clinical applications

A 55-year-old male presented with severe and advanced periodontal disease in his remaining mandibular teeth (Fig. 1). He had been informed about the hopeless prognosis of the mandibular teeth for many years, however his fear of dentistry prevented him from completing the recommended care. The seeding of bacteria as a consequence of the periodontal disease became a focus when other heart-related concerns were discovered. The patient was adamant in his desire to replace the teeth with a fixed prosthesis, as he did not think that he could tolerate anything removable. One of the reasons that he procrastinated about treatment was that he had been informed that the teeth were to be extracted, followed by a prolonged healing phase of approximately 4 months, implant placement, healing again followed by impressioning, and the prosthetic phase to complete treatment. The patient had not been made aware of any other alternative protocol for implant placement.

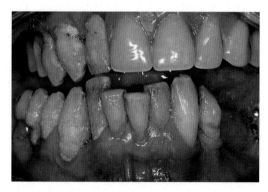

Fig. 1. Preoperative view of hopeless mandibular teeth.

Intraoral examination revealed extreme mobility, with many teeth being held in place by the formation of a thick calculus bridge. There was swollen and edematous tissue, loss of attachment, and bleeding upon probing (Fig. 2A, B). To facilitate the diagnosis, the patient was informed about the benefits of 3-D imaging to help determine the extent of remaining bone that would be necessary to allow support for a fixed restoration. The patient was informed that without CT scan imaging, it would be impossible to understand the bony topography or assess the location of vital structures such as the inferior alveolar nerve. The patient was educated in the benefits of advanced planning to avoid potential complications and to determine what treatment alternatives were possible, taking the guesswork out of the process. The patient agreed, and a CBCT scan was taken using a New-Tom 3G machine (AFP Imaging, Elmsford, NY.)

The scan was first evaluated using the machine's native software (NNT, AFP Imaging), and was then exported into a form that would make the data accessible to interactive treatment planning software applications. The DICOM data (Digital Imaging and Communications in Medicine) was then imported into SIMPlant (Materialise Dental, Glen Burnie, MD) for detailed assessment of the anatomy and evaluation of potential implant receptor sites. The SIMPlant software converts the CBCT scan data into four basic undistorted interactive views for clinical evaluation: (1) reconstructed panoramic view, (2) axial view, (3) cross-sectional view, and (4) the 3-D view. Precise planning can be accomplished only when all of these views fully appreciated.

The reconstructed panoramic image revealed a 2-dimensional assessment of the mandible and the remaining teeth (Fig. 3). The CBCT-generated panoramic view offers many benefits over conventional 2-D imaging with the interactivity of the software application. It is possible to scroll through the various panoramic images to help visualize the shape of the mandible and visualize the position of the teeth and path of the inferior alveolar nerve. It is also possible to change the gray-scale through a "windowing" of the CT scan data, which can also enhance the visualization of the anatomic

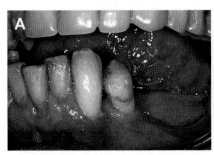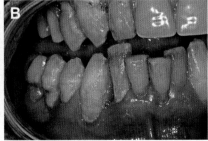

Fig. 2. (*A*) Left side reveals the severely resorbed posterior edentulous ridge. (*B*) Right side reveals the poor condition of the remaining teeth and gingival recession.

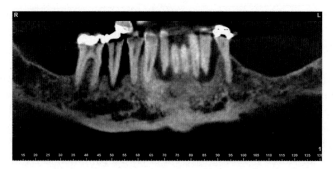

Fig. 3. Preoperative panoramic radiograph. Rampant bone loss is evident.

structures. However, the ultimate power of 3-D imaging is the ability to use all of the available tools to diagnose and construct a treatment plan properly. After a viewing the panoramic reconstructions, the cross-sectional or coronal views are carefully evaluated. Moving around the arch, the destructive process of advanced periodontal disease was evaluated with greater appreciation of the facial and lingual bone loss, which could not be detected through the either conventional or CBCT-reconstructed panoramic images (Fig. 4A–C).

Following the author's standard protocol, the next step was to determine the location of the right and left mental foramina. This was accomplished by carefully assessing the continuity of the buccal cortical plate in the axial view. By scrolling inferiorly to superiorly through each axial slice, the break in the cortical buccal or facial bone indicated the exit path of the inferior alveolar or mental nerve. Depending on the scanning protocol and the position and symmetry of the patient, the right and left mental foramina may not be evident in the same axial slice. Thus, the right and left side may need to be assessed separately. The mental foramina can be clearly seen in Fig. 5A. Once the bilateral foramina had been located, the path of the nerve was traced through the right and left posterior mandible. Planning implants in the anterior symphysis could then be accomplished, leaving an adequate zone of safety avoiding close proximity to the nerves (Fig. 5B).

Using the panoramic, axial, and cross-sectional images, five potential receptor sites were found between the mental foramina, and two posterior receptor sites were located on each side (Fig. 6). The removal of the remaining teeth in the anterior mandible would leave approximately 4 to 5 mm of residual alveolar crestal bone surrounding the postextraction sites. This bone was planned to be removed to gain adequate width of bone for immediate implant placement. Each placement was then individually confirmed in the cross-sectional images to ensure adequate bone volume surrounding the implant, and proper angulation, and position with regard the ultimate prosthetic reconstruction (Fig. 7A–E). The yellow extensions projecting from the coronal aspect of each implant represent the potential abutment

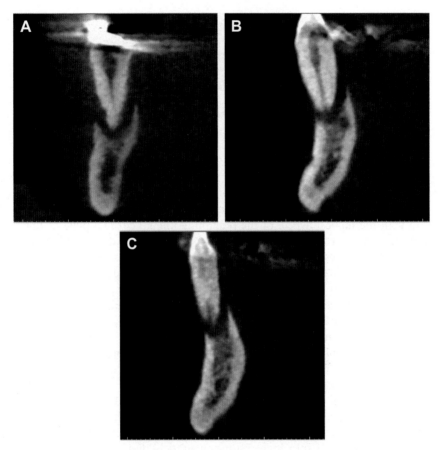

Fig. 4. (*A–C*) Cross-sectional CT scan slices reveal the significant loss of bone surrounding the remaining natural teeth.

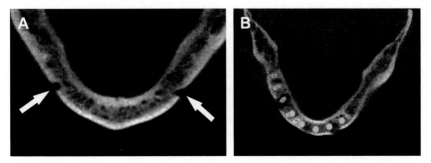

Fig. 5. (*A*) The axial image is important for the identification of the mental foramina as indicated by the arrows. (*B*) The space in the anterior symphysis was evaluated for the placement of five simulated implants.

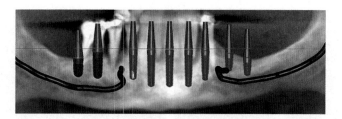

Fig. 6. After the mandibular nerve had been traced bilaterally, nine potential implant receptor sites were identified.

trajectories and are very useful in determining the relationship to the desired occlusion. The implants were specifically placed to gain adequate stabilization with the highest aspect of the remaining lingual cortical plate of bone, although some threads would be exposed on the facial. Additionally, visualization of other vessels (lingual) was noted to avoid potential complications (see Fig. 7A). This process was not arbitrary, simplistic, or accomplished without careful attention to detail. The planning phase however, was not complete at this stage. The final "tweaking" and ultimate confirmation were completed after case presentation to the patient. After presenting several treatment plan options to patient, it was determined that five implants placed in the symphysis area would provide adequate support for a fixed hybrid restoration while meeting the patient's needs (Fig. 8).

The opportunity to maximize the technological capabilities of CT/CBCT planning can only be realized when the 3-D dimensional reconstructed *virtual* models are used [5]. Using advanced segmentation modalities found in SIMPlant Pro, or SIMPlant Master software application, the existing data were converted into high-resolution models that can be rotated and viewed in any position on the computer screen (Fig. 9A). The bone and the teeth were separated by using 3-D masking tools providing a picture of the extraction sites that could not be visualized by any other means (see Fig. 9B). The ability to appreciate the bone topography in this manner cannot be underestimated. The lingual view of the existing teeth and mandible can be seen in Fig. 10. Using sophisticated masking tools allowed the remaining natural teeth to be "removed" from the 3-D model, to help visualize the positioning of the implants within the bony housing of the extraction sites, and enhance the capability to accurately assess proximity to the mental foramina (Fig. 11). Without masking, it would be difficult to properly assimilate all of the elements to finalize the plan (Fig. 12A). However, other tools can also aid in this process. The use of transparency enabled the implant abutment projections to be seen through the translucent teeth in Fig. 12B. Further application of the transparency effect can be very useful in appraising the parallelism of the implants and proximity to the path of the inferior alveolar nerve (see Fig. 12C). When the 3-D mandibular bone was removed entirely, the clinical crowns and root morphology

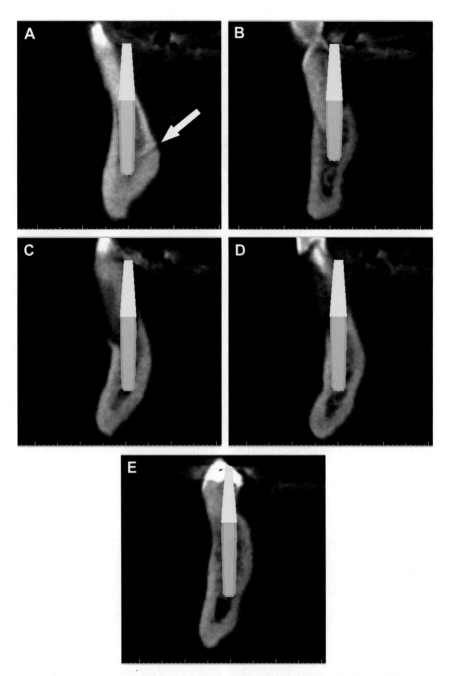

Fig. 7. (*A*) The simulated implant was placed within the anterior mandible in a position consistent with a screw-retained prosthesis. Note the lingual vessel (*arrow*). (*B–E*) Although there was significant bone loss, there was sufficient bone for to fixate the implants within the buccal and lingual cortical plates.

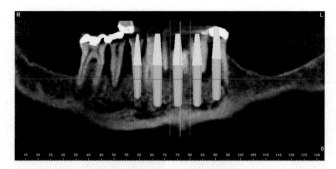

Fig. 8. The panoramic reconstruction reveals five evenly and parallel-placed simulated implants. Note that four of five were at the same vertical height.

were readily apparent (Fig. 13). An anterior loop of the right inferior alveolar nerve was noted and appreciated in finalizing the spatial position of the implants (see *arrow* in Fig. 13).

As previously discussed, the residual alveolar process was to be reduced after extraction of the remaining teeth. Using 3-D modeling enables a precise consideration of the bony site for proper reduction based on the needs of the reconstruction (Fig. 14A). Before virtually reducing the bone, the vertical positioning of the implants can be appreciated by visualizing the actual representation of realistic implants. The interactive software application contains a library of manufacturer-specific implants by type, diameter, and length. Many implant manufacturers have supplied CAD files for use in the software application, greatly enhancing the planning capability. For this case, five Tapered Screw-Vent implants (Zimmer Dental, Carlsbad, CA) were used. The actual realistic CAD implants were then used for final visualization revealing the shape, thread pattern, apical configuration, and internal aspect of the prosthetic connection. It is the author's contention that placing all implants parallel and at the same vertical position (if

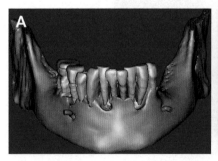
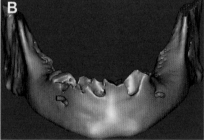

Fig. 9. (*A*) With advanced software segmentation techniques, the teeth and surrounding bone can be clearly seen in the 3-D reconstructed image. (*B*) Creating separate volumes allows the teeth to be virtually removed from the bone revealing the residual socket morphology.

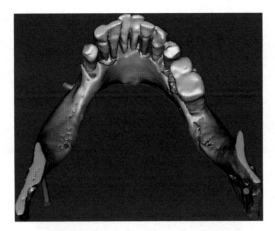

Fig. 10. The lingual-occlusal view of the mandibular complex.

possible), aids the prosthetic and laboratory phase of a screw-retained prosthesis. By removing the bone from the 3-D view, it was found that not all of
the implants were placed at the same vertical dimension (see Fig. 14B). Parallel placement was easily accomplished by use of the "paralleling" tool in
SIMPlant. Vertical "tweaking" was accomplished with the "translation"
tool, which can move the implant in very precise, small increments. Final
confirmation was achieved by slicing through the 3-D view to reveal the
bone, the implant, and the yellow abutment projection (Fig. 15).

When there is an edentulous mandible or maxilla, a radiopaque barium
sulfate template of a diagnostic wax-up or duplicate denture can be made
in advance to be worn during the CT scan process. This scanning or "scannographic" template can then help to determine the ideal position of the

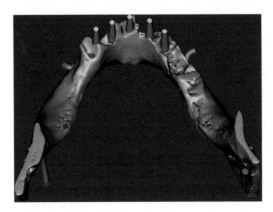

Fig. 11. With the teeth removed, the five implants were evaluated for placement with the aid of
yellow abutment projections.

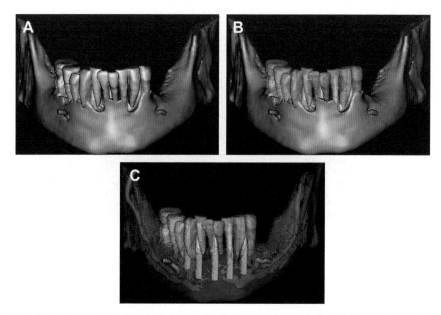

Fig. 12. (*A–C*) The relationship between the planned implants, the remaining teeth, and the underlying inferior alveolar nerve can be seen when the transparency tools are used.

teeth in relation to the underlying bone [6–10]. When existing teeth are present, as in this case presentation, this becomes more difficult. Therefore, a new tool (Virtual Teeth), originally envisioned by the author in early 1994, was recently introduced as a continually evolving application within SIMPlant to aid in assessing the restorative needs for any edentulous site, whether it be a single tooth or full arch. It is the author's contention that these interactive planning tools will play a significant future role for linking CT scan planning data to CAD/CAM applications [3,11].

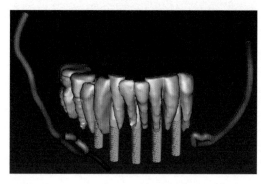

Fig. 13. Removing the bone entirely allows for careful assessment of implant placement within proximity of the nerves.

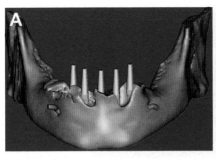
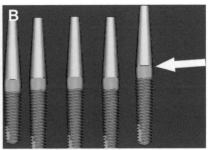

Fig. 14. (*A, B*) The simulated implants can be further examined within the confines of the residual alveolar ridge, and when the bone is removed, the implant-to-implant relationships can be fully appreciated. *Note:* This original plan (*B*) was modified to allow for all implants to be placed at the same vertical height (*arrow*).

Using the virtual tooth tool, a "virtual occlusion" was configured over the existing dentition allowing for a CAD representation of the desired tooth position (Fig. 16). The 3-D mandibular bone was also virtually "reduced" by 4 to 5 mm, and the vertical placement of the teeth was easily appreciated in all views (Fig. 17A, B). The use of CAD virtual teeth can help in assessing the final prosthesis design by helping to understand crown-to-root ratio, and the need for pink acrylic or porcelain flanges for lip support or cosmetics. The occlusal view of the 3-D mandible and virtual occlusion demonstrate this valuable prosthetic tool (Fig. 18A). The close-up view in Fig. 18B reveals the yellow abutment projections and their relationship

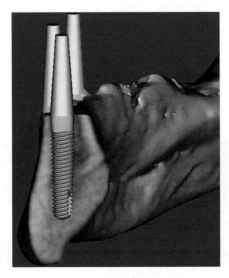

Fig. 15. Advanced 3-D segmentation tools allow for sectioning of the mandible, revealing the spatial position of the realistic implant and yellow abutment projection.

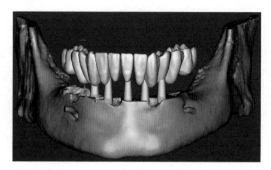

Fig. 16. The incorporation of a "virtual occlusion" helps in positioning the implants within the restorative envelope of the teeth.

with the occlusal scheme. By using these 3-D tools, the surgical and prosthetic team can easily assess the final proposed result before ever touching the scalpel to the patient, minimizing potential problems resulting from malpositioned implants (see Fig. 18C). In this manner, using all of the tools available, true *restoratively driven implant dentistry* can be accomplished. When the plan has been finalized, the data are sent via e-mail for fabrication of a bone-borne surgical template that will serve as the definitive guide for the placement of the implants (Materialise Dental, Lueven, Belgium).

Surgical intervention

Surgical templates have been fabricated in several forms: (1) the original bone-borne template, (2) the tooth-borne template, and, more recently, (3) a soft tissue–borne template. As this particular case presentation involved tooth extraction, bone reduction, and implant placement, it was elected to use a bone-borne template. There is an important caveat with regard to tooth extractions and alveolectomy when working with bone-borne templates: do not remove the bone until all osteotomies have been prepared. If the bone is modified before use of the template, it will no longer fit

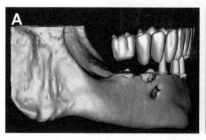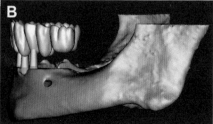

Fig. 17. (*A, B*) The right and left lateral 3-D reconstructions reveal the virtual teeth, and the occlusal plane in the posterior mandible.

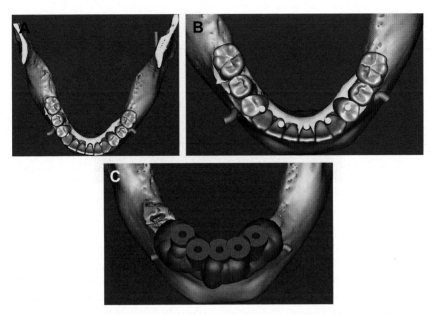

Fig. 18. (*A–C*) The occlusal views reveal the virtual teeth, the yellow abutment projections, and the preview of the surgical guide.

accurately to the underlying bone [5]. Tooth extractions should always be done atraumatically, taking care not to remove bone if possible. The bony foundation should remain intact to allow for stability and fit of the bone-borne template. Therefore, bone reduction is a step that follows the osteotomy preparation, not before. A technique that was not demonstrated for this case involves using a special "bone-reduction template" that can be fabricated through stereolithography to achieve a high level of accuracy when planning to place implants simultaneous to substantial vertical bone reduction in the anterior symphysis [12]. The extractions were performed and the soft granulation or cystic tissue was carefully removed (Fig. 19). Using the bone-borne templates, five osteotomies were drilled into the mandibular bone as per the CT scan. Once the osteotomies were prepared, the bone was leveled to achieve the anticipated dimension. Five tapered screw-vent implants were then successfully placed (Zimmer Dental, Carlsbad, California). Four of the implants with their attached fixture mounts demonstrate parallelism, with the fifth or middle implant at the desired vertical height of bone level to the lingual cortical plate (Fig. 20). Proper implant spacing, and the residual, remaining bone defects are evident in Fig. 21. Autogenous bone was collected from each site and mixed with mineralized bone to fill the defects to support the soft tissue. Collagen strips (Collacote, Zimmer Dental) were soaked in sterile saline solution and placed over the entire surgical site. Five titanium, direct-to-the implant, screw-receiving cylinders (Titan

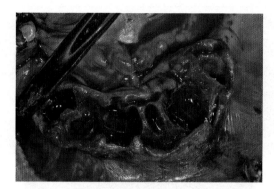

Fig. 19. The alveolar ridge after the teeth have been extracted.

Implants, Bergenfield, New Jersey) were attached to each implant, and the soft tissue approximated and sutured using 4-0 vicryl sutures.

Once the site had been sutured, a rectangular piece of rubber dam material with pre-punched holes was placed over each cylinder and adapted to the underlying soft tissue. A prefabricated prosthesis was placed over the cylinders, and cold-cure acrylic injected into horizontal holes to fixate the cylinders (Fig. 22A). The prosthesis was then removed to add and/or trim the acrylic (see Fig. 22B). Once polished, the prosthesis was screw-retained to the implants, and the bite adjusted (Figs. 23 and 24). The transitional prosthesis was fabricated as a duplicate of the original position of the patient's natural dentition. Postoperative instructions were given to the patient, with specific instructions as to use of a soft diet on the immediate load restoration. The patient returned after 2 weeks with normal healing, and report of little swelling or pain. All of the sutures were then removed, and the patient was followed for 8 weeks to monitor healing.

After 8 weeks, the transitional prosthesis was removed, and the underlying soft tissue evaluated for maturation and peri-implant sulcus depth

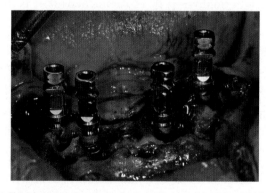

Fig. 20. Five parallel implants placed as per the software plan. The middle implant has the fixture mount removed.

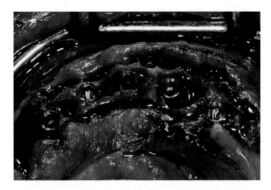

Fig. 21. The five implants placed within the residual extraction sockets as seen in the occlusal-lingual view.

(Fig. 25). Fixture mount impressions transfers were reattached for impressioning and to transpose the implant position to a working cast (Fig. 26). Using conventional prosthodontic protocols, a baseplate was fabricated with wax-rim for bite and vertical dimension registration. A complete denture set-up was fabricated and using two implants, screw-retained for stability and reproduction of the centric relation records. Once the bite was verified, and the esthetic desires of the patient satisfied, the denture set-up and working cast were ready to be sent to the dental laboratory for the fabrication of a CAD/CAM bar. One final step was necessary and essential: the verification of the master working cast. All of the transfer impression posts were indexed with resin (GC Pattern Resin, GC America Inc., Alsip, Illinois), and screw-retained intraorally to verify the fit against the master cast. The materials were all sent to the dental laboratory (York Dental Lab, Branford, Connecticut) for final processing and virtual design of the CAD/CAM bar.

The process for bar fabrication involved the optical scanning of both the master working cast and the completed denture wax-up. Various methodologies have been developed to achieve solid, one-piece CAD/CAM bars [12–18]. For this case, the digital information obtained through the optical

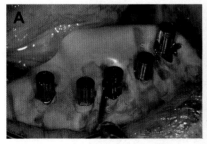
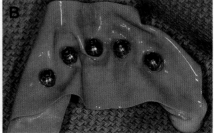

Fig. 22. (A, B) Titanium cylinders projecting from the implants and the protective rubber dam. The prosthesis and the rubber dam after removal.

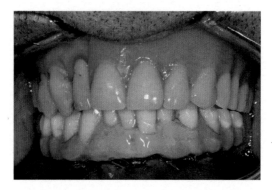

Fig. 23. The screw-retained fixed-hybrid prosthesis resembled the patient's original teeth.

scan allowed for CAD/CAM design using specialized software applications (ARCHITECH PSR, Biomet 3i, Palm Beach Gardens, FL). Before fabrication, the design specifications were sent via e-mail to the dental laboratory for inspection and approval (Fig. 27A–C). Using a computer numeric control (CNC) milling machine, the one-piece mandibular framework (CAM StructSURE Precision Milled Bar, Biomet 3i) was milled from a solid blank of titanium alloy. Unlike conventional protocols, the one-piece milled bar did not require additional components or abutments, as it fit directly to the implants with fixation screws (Fig. 28) [19,20]. The solid CAD/CAM bar fit passively onto the implants, and did not impinge upon the underlying soft tissue (Fig. 29). The occlusal view of the master cast with the CAD/CAM framework, seen in Fig. 30A, was then verified intraorally in Fig. 30B. CAD/CAM technology was significant in reducing the labor associated with traditional bar fabrication, since the entire design process was completed virtually. CAD/CAM milling also reduces problems inherent with lost-wax casting methods, soldering or welding, passive fit, and reducing the number of parts since separate, individual abutments were not required [16–20]. Once passive fit had been established, the laboratory

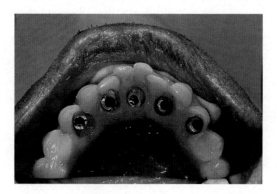

Fig. 24. The screw-access holes can been seen in the occlusal view.

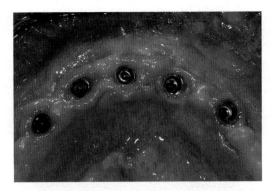

Fig. 25. The healed site shows the expanded zone of attached gingival tissue.

completed the denture wax-up using conventional protocols after applying a silicone index of the desired tooth position (Fig. 31A, B).

The final prosthesis was processed as a fixed-hybrid screw-retained restoration using pink acrylic to simulate interdental papilla, minimize air flow under the prosthesis, and support the lower lip (Fig. 32). The 3-D planning allowed for parallel implants and screw access holes to be placed in strategic positions that were easily obturated and camouflaged (Fig. 33). The use of CT scan imaging, interactive treatment planning software with CAD capabilities, and precise placement tools enabled excellent presurgical prosthetic planning that simulated all aspects of the case before the scalpel ever touched the patient. Therefore, it was possible to accomplish simultaneous tooth extractions with parallel implant placement guided by CT-derived templates, and delivery of an immediate transitional restoration that allowed the patient to leave with a fixed restoration on the day of surgery. After adequate healing, and an evaluation of the surgical accuracy, the ability to create a CAD/CAM milled titanium bar was enhanced, while decreasing

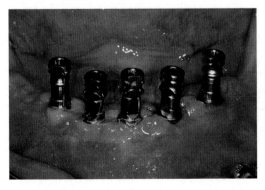

Fig. 26. Fixture level transfer impression posts placed on the implants and ready for the impression phase.

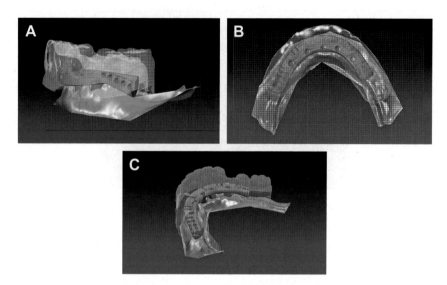

Fig. 27. (*A–C*) The virtual CAD restoration can be seen in various views within the outline of the restorative envelope.

both laboratory and clinician chair time, reducing the number of parts, therefore reducing certain associated costs. The final fixed restoration met the functional and esthetic needs of the patient (Fig. 34).

Computer-aided design planning capabilities

Presurgical prosthetic planning for placement and restoration of dental implants should follow a sound foundation of accepted prosthodontic protocols. The importance of accurate study casts, determination of vertical dimension of occlusion, proper articulation, diagnostic wax-ups, lip support,

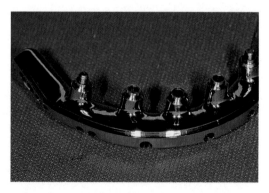

Fig. 28. The solid milled CAD/CAM bar allows a direct connection to the implant without need for additional abutments.

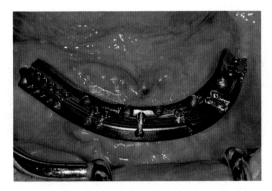

Fig. 29. The passive fit verified intraorally.

and an understanding of the functional and esthetic concerns cannot be underestimated to achieve predictable results. To facilitate accurate planning, it is desirable to create a radiopaque template that demonstrates the position of the proposed restoration with a diagnostic wax-up or a laboratory-fabricated duplicate of the patient's denture. Incorporating a radiopaque material such as barium sulfate into an acrylic diagnostic appliance turns it into a scanning or *scannographic* template to be worn by the patient during the acquisition of the CT scan image, a technique that has been well documented [2,4,6–10,12,21]. Thus, the position of the desired occlusion and tooth position as it relates to the underlying bone can be fully appreciated in various CT scan images. Therefore, digital technology has provided clinicians with new tools to go beyond conventional stone and wax.

For a fully edentulous patient, a duplicate of the patient's existing denture was fabricated using a Lang Denture Duplicator (Lang Dental Mfg Co., Inc., Wheeling, Illinois). Using a mixture of 20% barium sulfate to 80% clear acrylic, a scannographic appliance was fabricated and used during the CT scan process. The 3-D reconstructed view of the patient's mandible with the radiopaque appliance can be seen in Fig. 35. Using CAD

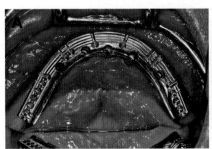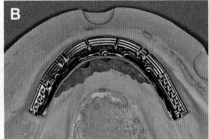

Fig. 30. (*A, B*) The occlusal view intraorally, and on the working cast indicates the screw-access holes of the implants, and the grooves for the labial silicone index.

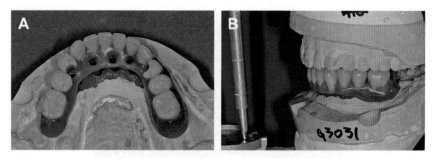

Fig. 31. (*A, B*) Using the silicone index, the teeth were positioned over the bar for a wax try-in.

masking and segmentation tools (SIMPlant Pro, Materialise Dental), the prosthesis can be virtually "separated" from the underlying bone. The scanning prosthesis represents the teeth and the flange extensions as they sit on the soft tissue (Fig. 36A, B). The prosthesis can be rotated so that the intaglio surface can be fully appreciated. Other methods to achieve similar results require a "dual-scan" technique where the patient is first scanned with the appliance in place, and then a second scan is completed of the appliance alone. To facilitate the process, special fiduciary markers incorporated in the scanning appliance allow for the two separate scan datasets to be "merged" together in the software application [4,8,9]. Regardless of the method, the ability to combine the desired 3-D restorative outcome with the underlying bony anatomy empowers the clinician with the necessary information to make educated decisions in determining the definitive plan of treatment.

The cross-sectional 2-D slice, which incorporates a radiopaque scanning template, revealed the relationship of the tooth position, occlusion, and flange extensions to the underlying bone (Fig. 37A). A simulated implant can then be placed and evaluated according to the author's "Triangle of Bone" (TOB) concept originally published in 1995 [22]. The TOB designates

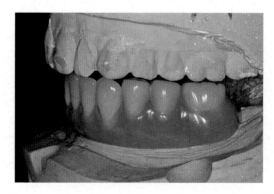

Fig. 32. Lateral view of the definitive prosthesis on the articulator.

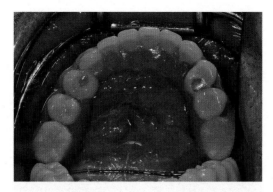

Fig. 33. The occlusal intraoral view of the definitive prosthesis.

a "zone" of available bone volume for a given implant receptor site as an aid in the decision process of determining proper implant placement [3,23]. As previously demonstrated, the trajectory of the implant can be better appreciated when an abutment projection (*yellow*) is extended through the prosthesis (see Fig. 37B). However, it is important that the planning phase continue, as more information is essential to ensure that each site is properly evaluated [3,23,24]. Using advanced software design tools, the mandible and the template can be visualized and "sliced" in the 3-D view allowing for unprecedented planning capabilities (Fig. 38A). The use of real CAD implants serves as a major advance in the interactive software application for implant planning. Choosing a specific type of implant (Astra Tech Inc., Waltham, Massachusetts) from the manufacturer's library improves visualization and positioning (see Fig. 38B). The abutment projection allows for determination of trajectory of the implant as it emerges through the prosthesis (see Fig. 38C). Until recently, this was the only tool that helped to link the restoration to the implant. Participating implant manufacturers provided the necessary CAD files to incorporate realistic implants, and then added files

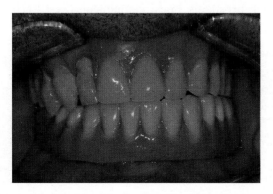

Fig. 34. A retracted view of the fixed-hybrid, screw-retained prosthesis.

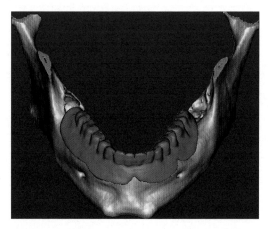

Fig. 35. An essential part of planning edentulous cases is the radiopaque scanning appliance, which can be separated from the bone on the 3-D reconstruction through computer software.

for virtual abutments as an extension of the implant library as incorporated into SIMPlant's Version 10 and 11.

When clinicians plan to place an implant and wish to place an abutment, there are now new choices that go beyond a schematic abutment projection. Realistic stock implant abutments can be selected based on shape, tissue cuff height, diameter, and purpose as seen in Fig. 39A. In the cross-sectional 3-D view, the implant can be placed in the desired position, and a realistic manufacturer-specific virtual abutment chosen based on the restorative needs of the site (Fig. 39B). The screw-receiving abutment connection (Uniabutment, Astra Tech Inc.) can be fully visualized as it engages the implant, and positioned with respect to the prosthesis, bone, and gingival, aiding the clinician in selecting the appropriate tissue cuff height (see Fig. 39C). Other realistic off-the-shelf stock abutments can be chosen when appropriate, and can assist in providing additional treatment options for the patient, quickly and efficiently. If one of the treatment options were to include an implant supported removable prosthesis, Locator abutments (Zest Anchors, Escondido,

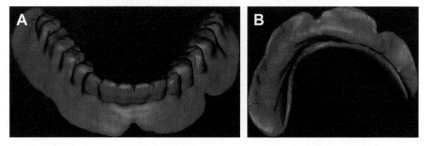

Fig. 36. (*A, B*) The scanning prosthesis as seen from the occlusal and intaglio view.

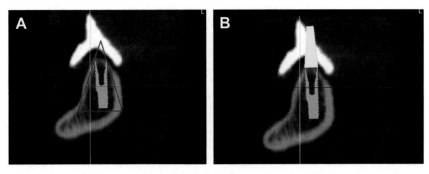

Fig. 37. (A, B) The cross-sectional allows for precise planning of the implant in relation to the radiopaque prosthesis and within the "Triangle of Bone".

CA) may be the abutment of choice (Fig. 40A). However, these abutments come in several different tissue cuff heights. The ability to place a realistic CAD abutment onto the implant helps clinicians to provide the correct component for the site, and in determining the parts required to complete a given restoration. A locator abutment can be virtually placed and evaluated in both the 2-D and 3-D views (see Fig. 40B). The frontal view of the mandible with all of the implants in place and "fitted" with the virtual locator abutments, can be more fully appreciated by applying the transparency effect to

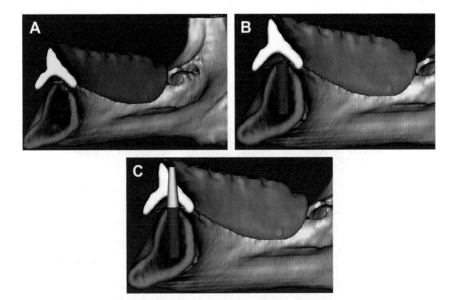

Fig. 38. (A–C) Virtual "slicing" of the 3-D reconstruction allows an unparalleled view as an aid to positioning the implant in the desired position in relation to the restorative needs of the patient.

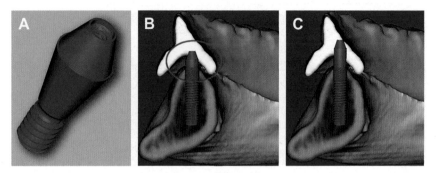

Fig. 39. (*A–C*) A realistic screw-receiving abutment can be chosen for the realistic implant (AstraTech), and a proper tissue cuff height can be established.

further judge the implant-to-implant placement, proximity to the mental foramina, and to evaluate vertical height position (Fig. 41A, B). These interactive software tools are indispensable for virtual planning. The occlusal view of the mandible with four implants and four locator abutments can be seen in Fig. 41C. The bony exostosis of the anterior mandible is dramatically apparent in this view and confirmed by viewing previously described cross-sectional slices.

Present and future CAD-CAM applications

The advent of realistic CAD implants, realistic CAD abutments, and virtual teeth allows for premier planning capabilities right now. This technology however has also proven to be a direct path to the future [3,11]. There are several companies currently developing new and exciting methods to

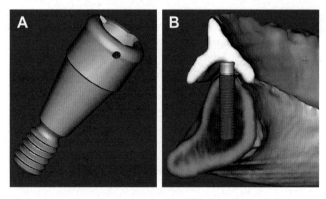

Fig. 40. (*A, B*) A removable option can be explored by choosing a realistic locator abutment attachment.

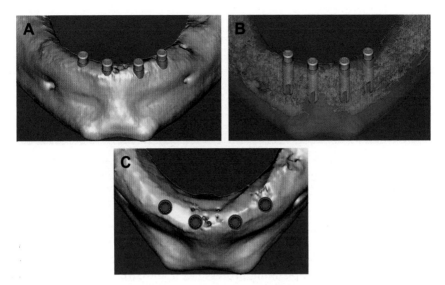

Fig. 41. (A–C) The position of four implants to accommodate a removable design with locator attachments can be fully appreciated in the 3-D reconstruction views.

harness digital dentistry through the use of intraoral optical scans, flash-CT scanning of impressions, laser-scanning of casts or impressions, and advanced CAD/CAM machining of both titanium and Zirconia materials [25–40]. It is the author's contention that dentistry will eventually move away from stone casts to a totally virtual world, eliminating conventional impressions in favor of optical or laser scanning technology [3,5,24].

For a single tooth application, many clinicians might think a CT/CBCT scan to be inappropriate. However, when a patient undergoes a CT/CBCT scan the 3-D reconstruction yields important information about the existing dentition, bone topography, and adjacent root morphology. With a single missing tooth, the technology exists to provide a "virtual" tooth to help provide the essential elements that guide the eventual positioning of the implant. Using CT cross-sectional slices, axial sections, the implant position could be established within the zone of the TOB, and confirmed with a "virtual" lateral incisor created to aid in determining the desired implant trajectory and emergence profile (Fig. 42A). The next step could allow for a virtual "stock" abutment to be placed onto the implant to evaluate the proposed position within the envelope of the tooth to be restored, in relation to the existing bony topography (see Fig. 42B). The final evaluation step is perhaps the most important. Interactive software applications have the power to strip away the surrounding bone to allow for careful inspection of the adjacent root morphology (Fig. 43A). The proximity of the implant can then be evaluated along the entire length of each root to avoid any potential complication. Additionally, the abutment itself can be evaluated for

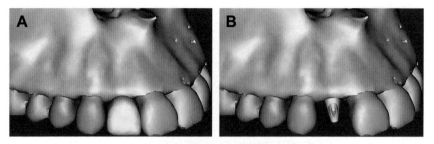

Fig. 42. (*A, B*) For a single missing lateral incisor, 3-D imaging is an essential tool to visualize bone and nearby vital structures. A virtual tooth is used to help plan proper implant positioning.

proximity to the tooth, to ensure that there is enough room to maintain interproximal contacts, and allow for healthy interdental papilla. Evaluating the implant without the abutment fails to provide all of the necessary information to complete the planning process (see Fig. 43B).

Using the "clipping" function in SIMPlant, it is possible to slice through the 3-D reconstruction, including the bone and the virtual tooth to inspect the implant trajectory, confirm the placement within the zone of the most volume of bone as defined by the TOB, and establish the desired emergence profile of the abutment (see Fig. 43C). If the stock abutment meets the needs for the site, then the part can be ordered from the implant manufacturer,

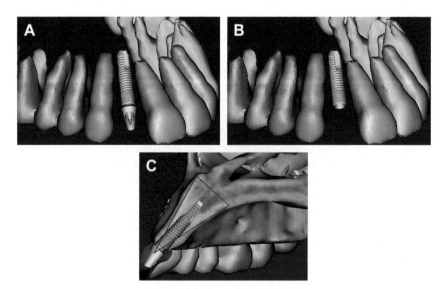

Fig. 43. (*A–C*) Removing the surrounding bone affords unprecedented views of the adjacent tooth roots. A realistic implant and abutment can be visualized in the 3-D cross-sectional image within the TOB.

diminishing inventory, while helping to improve cost estimates for the restorative phase well in advance of the treatment. Thus it is possible to provide very accurate plans that include both the surgical and restorative aspects of the treatment to be rendered to the patient. Once formulated, the CT scan data set will be used to fabricate a surgical guide, linking the virtual plan to the surgical intervention.

When a stock abutment is not appropriate because of various reasons, clinicians usually turn to custom or patient-specific abutments. The usual process involves intraoral impressioning the site to transfer the location of the implant to a master stone cast. The dental laboratory technician would then create a diagnostic study cast, fabricate a wax-up, and then invest and cast the wax pattern according to the conventions of the lost-wax casting method. Recent technologies allow for CAD/CAM design and milling, which provides a more accurate, cost-effective, efficient, and consistent product [41–43]. The use of computer-milled abutments by individual clinicians and dental laboratories has increased dramatically in the past few years; however, a standard impression phase is still required. New

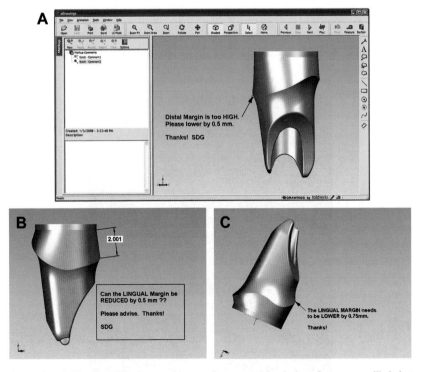

Fig. 44. (A–C) The virtual implant position can be exported for design of a custom-milled abutment. Using a 3-D viewing software application facilitates communication between the lab and the clinician, allowing for appropriate changes to be made.

technology allows for an abutment to be fabricated directly from the CT scan data, without the need for impressions or stone casts. Using the interactive software applications combined with CAD/CAM technologies, it has become possible to create a *virtual* abutment on a *virtual implant,* which better meets the morphology required to establish the ideal foundation for the ultimate tooth restoration. While not commercially available when this article was written, the ability to go from scan to virtual abutment has been done, and will hopefully be made available in the near future [3,11].

Once the scan has been taken, and the plan completed, a special stereolithographic data file (STL) is exported for use in the abutment CAD design process. Using specialized 3-D software applications, the abutment design can be sent through the Internet with a 3-D viewer to allow the laboratory or the clinician to review, evaluate, and comment. Fig. 44A shows a virtual abutment within the 3-D viewing software (SolidWorks Corporation, Concord, MA) showing comments made by the author. The viewing software allows for the user to make measurements and add comments, which would then be sent back to the design team (Fig. 44B). The abutment can be rotated in any position, with zooming capabilities for more precise visualization of areas of specific interest (see Fig. 44C). Once completed, the final CAD/CAM designed abutment can be sent back for incorporation into the implant planning software for final inspection and approval (Fig. 45). Therefore, the technology exists to go from a CT scan to a virtual implant, and a patient-specific virtual abutment, which can then be sent to a CNC

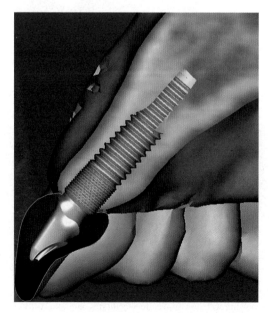

Fig. 45. An ideal virtual abutment simulated on a realistic implant within a virtual tooth.

milling machine for fabrication from either titanium or zirconia. The next logical step would be to virtually fabricate the coping, or final crown, which would sit on the abutment. The future is now.

Summary

CT and CBCT technology provides clinicians with new methods to view patient anatomy exceeding conventional 2-D radiology. Interactive software applications allow for improved interpretation of the CT scan data by incorporating tools for identifying vital anatomy, bone topography and quality, simulated implant placement, simulated abutment placement, and the fabrication of CT-derived surgical templates. The use of realistic CAD implants and CAD abutments provides the clinician with unprecedented abilities to accurately link the implant placement to the bone, and the ultimate restoration. Thus, the emergence of CT-based guided surgical protocols have created new and often dramatic treatment alternatives that could not be accomplished without 3-D imaging technologies. However, the scan is only one part of the equation, which is why the author contends that "It's not the SCAN, it's the PLAN" when applying this technology in everyday clinical practice.

Proper use of this new technology must be based on a solid foundation of fundamental surgical and prosthodontic protocols. Advances in software and associated hardware have empowered clinicians with the necessary tools to harness the technology, while remaining true to conventional standards. Using a scanning appliance during image acquisition places the desired restoration onto the bone for evaluation and site assessment for dental implants. This essential step helps to link the restorative requirements with the surgical intervention before ever touching the scalpel to the patient. The ability to create a "virtual occlusion" can further enhance both the diagnostic phase, and the fabrication of a CT-derived surgical guide. Combining improved diagnostics allows for better placement of the implants, which facilitates the restorative phase. When multiple implants are desired and can be surgically placed accurately and parallel, there is a greater potential to fabricate a passive fit of the prosthesis. Even with enhanced interactive CT software treatment plans, an impression phase is still required to fabricate a CAD/CAM milled bar as previously illustrated.

Accuracy of the 3-D planning phase will soon evolve with improved tools to communicate directly with laboratory-based milling machines, maximizing the ability to create CAD/CAM implant restorations similar to the innovations of the CEREC 3D system (Sirona, Patterson Dental Co, Milwaukee, WI) with intraoral optical scanning and milling for individual tooth restorations. Emerging technologies have been developed based on laser scanning technology referred to as "parallel confocal" light theory, which creates an electronic impression of a prepared tooth via a hand-held intraoral device (iTero, Caden, Inc., Carlstadt, NJ). Recently introduced, the E4D Dentist chairside solution does not require any reflective powdering agent for their IOD (IntraOral Digitizer) laser-optical scanning process for creating digital impressions of tooth preparations (D4D Technologies, LLC, Richardson, TX).

It has been demonstrated that computer-milled patient specific abutments (Atlantis, Astra Dental, Waltham, MA) can be milled from an STL file of a realistic CAD implant exported from an interactive software application (SIMPlant) without intraoral impressioning or stone casts [3]. As manufacturer-specific CAD files have now been incorporated into libraries of data that can be manipulated within the framework of the virtual world of 3-D CT scan imaging, it is postulated that this technology will gain momentum as the dental implant manufactures realize the future potential of combining CT scan technology, virtual implant planning, guided surgery, and CAD/CAM manufacturing of implant supported restorations. The enhanced capability of innovative software applications that allow clinicians to interpret and maneuver through various 3-D images has far-reaching implications when interactive treatment planning software is combined with CAD and manufacturing. Using all of the available virtual tools, true *restoratively driven implant dentistry* can be accomplished, ultimately benefiting our patients.

References

[1] Ganz SD. CT scan technology: an evolving tool for predictable implant placement and restoration. Int Mag Oral Implantol 2001;1:6–13.
[2] Ganz SD. Presurgical planning with CT-derived fabrication of surgical guides. J Oral Maxillofac Surg 2005;63(9 Suppl 2):59–71.
[3] Ganz SD. Defining new paradigms for assessment of implant receptor sites—the use of CT/CBCT and interactive virtual treatment planning for congenitally missing lateral incisors. Compend Contin Educ Dent 2008;29(5):256–67.
[4] Balshi SF, Wolfinger GJ, Balshi TJ. Surgical planning and prosthesis construction using computed tomography, CAD/CAM technology, and the Internet for immediate loading of dental implants. Int J Periodontics Restorative Dent 2006;26(3):239–47.
[5] Ganz SD. Use of stereolithographic models as diagnostic and restorative aids for predictable immediate loading of implants. Pract Proced Aesthet Dent 2003;15(10):763–71.
[6] Marchack CB, Moy PK. The use of a custom template for immediate loading with the definitive prosthesis: a clinical report. J Calif Dent Assoc 2003;31(12):925–9.
[7] Tardieu PB, Vrielinck L, Escolano E. Computer-assisted implant placement. A case report: treatment of the mandible. Int J Oral Maxillofac Implants 2003;18(4):599–604.
[8] Marchack CB. An immediately loaded CAD/CAM-guided definitive prosthesis: a clinical report. J Prosthet Dent 2005;93(1):8–12.
[9] Sherry JS, Sims LO, Balshi SF. A simple technique for immediate placement of definitive engaging custom abutments using computerized tomography and flapless guided surgery. Quintessence Int 2007;38(9):755–62.
[10] Marchack CB. CAD/CAM-guided implant surgery and fabrication of an immediately loaded prosthesis for a partially edentulous patient. J Prosthet Dent 2007;97(6):389–94.

[11] Ganz SD. "Using stereolithographic CT technology for immediate functional and non-functional loading". Presented at the Annual Meeting of the Academy of Osseointegration. Orlando, Florida, March 12, 2005.

[12] Ganz SD. Techniques for the use of CT imaging for the fabrication of surgical guides. Atlas Oral Maxillofac Surg Clin North Am 2006;14(1):75–97.

[13] Ortorp A, Jemt T. Clinical experiences of computer numeric control-milled titanium frameworks supported by implants in the edentulous jaw: a 5-year prospective study. Clin Implant Dent Relat Res 2004;6(4):199–209.

[14] Hjalmarsson L, Smedberg JI. A 3-year retrospective study of Cresco frameworks: preload and complications. Clin Dent Relat Res 2005;7(4):189–99.

[15] Mitrani R, Vasilic M, Bruguera A. Fabrication of an implant-supported reconstruction utilizing CAD/CAM technology. Pract Proced Aesthet Dent 2005;17(1):71–8 [quiz 80].

[16] Ehrenkranz H, Langer B, Marotta L. Complete-arch maxillary rehabilitation using a custom-designed and manufactured titanium framework: a clinical report. J Prosthet Dent 2008;99(1):8–13.

[17] Jemt T, Henry P, Lindén B, et al. Implant-supported laser-welded titanium and conventional cast frameworks in the partially edentulous law: a 5-year prospective multicenter study. Int J Prosthodont 2003;16(4):415–21.

[18] Brudvik JS, Chigurupati K. The milled implant bar: an alternative to spark erosion. J Can Dent Assoc 2002;68(8):485–8.

[19] Drago CJ. Two new clinical/laboratory protocols for CAD/CAM implant restorations. J Am Dent Assoc 2006;137(6):794–800.

[20] Drago CJ, Peterson T. Treatment of an edentulous patient with CAD/CAM technology: a clinical report. J Prosthodont 2007;16(3):200–8.

[21] Sanna AM, Molly L, van Steenberghe D. Immediately loaded CAD-CAM manufactured fixed complete dentures using flapless implant placement procedures: a cohort study of consecutive patients. J Prosthet Dent 2007;97(6):331–9.

[22] Ganz SD. The triangle of bone—a formula for successful implant placement and restoration. The Implant Society, Inc 1995;5(5):2–6.

[23] Ganz SD. The reality of anatomy and the triangle of bone. Inside Dentistry. 2006;2(5): 72–7.

[24] Ganz SD. CT-derived model-based surgery for immediate loading of maxillary anterior implants. Pract Proced Aesthet Dent 2007;19(5):311–8 [quiz 320, 302].

[25] Osorio J. Use of the Atlantis abutment in restorative practice speeds time to function and aesthetics [Interview]. Dent Implantol Update 2000;11(8):57–62.

[26] Kerstein RB, Castellucci F, Osorio J. Ideal gingival form with computer-generated permanent healing abutments. Compend Contin Educ Dent 2000;21(10):793–7, 800–801.

[27] Kucey BK, Fraser DC. The Procera abutment—the fifth generation abutment for dental implants. J Can Dent Assoc 2000;66(8):445–9.

[28] Luthardt RG, Sandkuhl O, Herold V, et al. Accuracy of mechanical digitizing with a CAD/CAM system for fixed restorations. Int J Prosthodont 2001;14(2):146–51.

[29] Schneider A, Kurtzman GM. Computerized milled solid implant abutments utilized at second stage surgery. Gen Dent 2001;49(4):416–20.

[30] Garg AK. The Atlantis components abutment: simplifying the tooth implant procedure. Dent Implantol Update 2002;13(9):65–70.

[31] Lang LA, Sierraalta M, Hoffensperger M, et al. Evaluation of the precision of fit between the Procera custom abutment and various implant systems. Int J Oral Maxillofac Implants 2003; 18(5):652–8.

[32] Ganz SD. Computer-milled patient-specific abutments: incredible quality with unprecedented simplicity. Pract Proced Aesthet Dent 2003;15(8 Suppl):37–44.

[33] Tselios N, Parel SM, Jones JD. Immediate placement and immediate provisional abutment modeling in anterior single-tooth implant restorations using a CAD/CAM application: a clinical report. J Prosthet Dent 2006;95(3):181–5.

[34] Quaas S, Rudolph H, Luthardt RG. Direct mechanical data acquisition of dental impressions for the manufacturing of CAD/CAM restorations. J Dent 2007;35(12): 903–8.

[35] Vafiadis DC. Computer-generated abutments using a coded healing abutment: a two-year preliminary report. Pract Proced Aesthet Dent 2007;19(7):443–8.

[36] Allum SR. Immediately loaded full-arch provisional implant restorations using CAD/CAM and guided placement: maxillary and mandibular case reports. Br Dent J 2008;204(7): 377–81.

[37] Piwowarczyk A, Ottl P, Lauer HC, et al. A clinical report and overview of scientific studies and clinical procedures conducted on the 3M ESPE Lava All-Ceramic System. J Prosthodont 2005;14(1):39–45.

[38] Priest G. Virtual-designed and computer-milled implant abutments. J Oral Maxillofac Surg 2005;63(9 Suppl 2):22–32.

[39] Vigolo P, Fonzi F, Majzoub Z, et al. An in vitro evaluation of titanium, zirconia, and alumina procera abutments with hexagonal connection. Int J Oral Maxillofac Implants 2006; 21(4):575–80.

[40] Grossmann Y, Pasciuta M, Finger IM. A novel technique using a coded healing abutment for the fabrication of a CAD/CAM titanium abutment for an implant-supported restoration. J Prosthet Dent 2006;95(3):258–61.

[41] Calderini A, Maiorana C, Garlini G, et al. A simplified method to assess precision of fit between framework and supporting implants: a preliminary study. Int J Oral Maxillofac Implants 2007;22(5):831–8.

[42] Ganz SD, Desai N, Weiner S. Marginal integrity of direct and indirect castings for implant abutments. Int J Oral Maxillofac Implants 2006;21(4):593–9.

[43] Witkowski S, Komine F, Gerds T. Marginal accuracy of titanium copings fabricated by casting and CAD/CAM techniques. J Prosthet Dent 2006;96(1):47–52.

ELSEVIER
SAUNDERS

THE DENTAL
CLINICS
OF NORTH AMERICA

Dent Clin N Am 52 (2008) 809–823

Cone-Beam CT: Applications in Orthodontics

Steven L. Hechler, DDS, MS

12800 Metcalf Avenue, Suite 1, Overland Park, KS 66213, USA

Orthodontists have routinely treated patients' malocclusions by applying forces in all three planes of space. The movement of alveolar bone may be accomplished in two directions: in a transverse direction, using a rapid maxillary expansion appliance, or in a sagittal direction, using a headgear or Herbst appliance. Tooth movement alone may also be accomplished using archwires and elastics, as evidenced by the vertical movement of teeth using vertical or box interarch elastics. For years, these three-dimensional (3D) movements have been diagnosed and treatment planned based on two-dimensional (2D) imaging. Cephalometric, panoramic, and periapical radiographs are a few of the 2D radiographs routinely used in orthodontic planning. Although these images have been the standard of care and are useful in assessing skeletal and dental relationships, their 2D diagnostic information can leave some questions unanswered in selected cases. This article discusses the application of cone-beam CT (CBCT) in various orthodontic tasks, from simple to more advanced. It also takes a glimpse into the future to determine how CBCT may become a normal part of high-tech orthodontic treatment.

Common diagnostic radiographs

Cephalometric radiology was introduced to orthodontics in 1931 by Broadbent in the United States and Hofrath in Germany. They developed standardized methods for obtaining these radiographs using cephalostats to facilitate reproducible head positioning for films taken at different time points [1]. These cephalometric radiographs are heavily relied on by orthodontists today to measure angular and linear dimensions using various anatomic landmarks. "Cephalometric" images constructed from CBCT

E-mail address: hechler@hechler.com

0011-8532/08/$ - see front matter © 2008 Elsevier Inc. All rights reserved.
doi:10.1016/j.cden.2008.05.001
dental.theclinics.com

scans have been shown to be as accurate as, or in some cases more accurate than, conventional 2D lateral cephalometric radiographs [2]. Additionally, lateral cephalometric radiographs constructed from the CBCT scans can use the information from the right and/or left half of the skull. Constructing these images using one half of the skull can overcome the problem faced with superimposition of the right and left ramus, body, molars, and mandibular condyles.

The panoramic radiograph was first proposed and experimented with in the 1930s by Dr. H. Numata of Japan. In the mid-1940s, the father of panoramic radiography, Dr. Yrjo Veli Paatero of Finland, refined the panoramic technique [3]. Since then, 2D panoramic radiography has been further refined and brought to a level previously unattained. The images made with these modern digital panoramic machines are clear and diagnostic; however, positioning errors and arch and teeth variations may have an effect on diagnostic efficacy. CBCT scans allow an infinite number of focal troughs to be specified and reformatted, compensating for arch variations. Also, separate "panoramic" radiographs can be obtained from the CBCT data, focusing on the maxillary arch and the mandible. Linear and angular dimensions have been shown to be more accurate using the CBCT panoramic images, compared with traditional panoramic radiographs, which is also true when viewing the condyles [4].

Several other views, projectional and tomographic, are used in orthodontics, but not as frequently. Most of these images can be reconstructed from the CBCT data if a CBCT scan has been acquired.

The contribution of CBCT in various diagnostic tasks is discussed in the following paragraphs.

Impacted canines

Possibly the most recognized need for CBCT imaging in orthodontics is that of impacted canine evaluation. The prevalence of impacted maxillary canines is approximately 0.9% to 3.0% [5,6]. The ratio of palatal to labial impactions has been shown to be as high as 9:1 [7]. Studies have been carried out relating the position of the impacted canine to the success of uncovery and orthodontic traction [8–10].

In the past, orthodontists have used the tube shift technique to compare two periapical radiographs taken at different beam angles to determine the facial/lingual position of the impacted canine. This same lingual, opposite buccal rule is helpful in determining whether the impacted canine is labial or lingual to the incisor roots; however, the degree of displacement is difficult to determine. CBCT imaging is precise in determining not only the labial/lingual relationship but also a more exact angulation of the impacted canine. These 3D images are beneficial in determining the proximity of adjacent incisor and premolar roots, which can be invaluable in determining the ease of uncovering and bonding and the vector of force that should be used to move the tooth into the arch with a lesser chance of adjacent root resorption.

A standard periapical radiograph of an impacted maxillary left canine (#11) is shown in Fig. 1A. This single film gives limited information about canine position or possible adjacent root resorption. The palatal location of the canine is obvious in the axial view of the CBCT scan using Dolphin 3D (Dolphin Imaging and Management Solutions, Chatsworth, California), in Fig. 1B. A view of the proximity of the canine to the central incisor (#9) is shown in the CBCT sagittal transparent hard tissue image in Fig. 1C. The two teeth are not in contact with one another, and no resorption is evident on the central incisor. A different type of image using the same Dolphin 3D software and CBCT data package is seen in Fig. 1D. This view shows the much closer relationship of the same canine to the adjacent lateral incisor (#10). No root resorption is obvious in the images. The uncovery, bonding, and direction of force vector for #11 is enhanced significantly by the knowledge supplied to the oral surgeon and orthodontist.

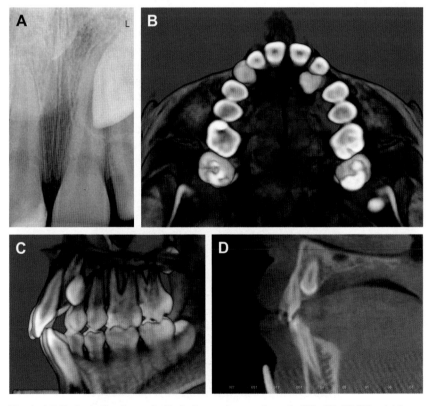

Fig. 1. (*A*) Periapical radiograph displaying an impacted tooth #11. (*B*) CBCT axial image showing the palatal position of tooth #11. (*C*) CBCT image of the relationship between teeth # 9 and #11. (*D*) Sagittal CBCT image displaying the proximity of #11 to the root of #10.

One should note that the four views in Fig. 1 are all static images made from a 3D CBCT scan. Using software like Dolphin 3D, the doctor can rotate the 3D skull, allowing for cuts at various angles to aid in visualization. The plane of view can be moved through the entire skull in all three axes of space. Some clinicians are now suggesting that tissue and bony uncovery of the significantly palatally displaced and impacted canines without orthodontic traction would allow these teeth to drift into the oral cavity spontaneously; they then may be bonded some months later by the orthodontist [11]. The enhanced knowledge of canine position supplied by the CBCT scans will aid the orthodontist as he or she determines whether to simply uncover the palatally impacted canine or apply immediate traction.

Other impacted teeth

Various other teeth become impacted less often than canines but still pose a significant orthodontic challenge. Maxillary central incisors can be impacted and displaced subsequent to the presence of a mesiodens. Fig. 2 shows a CBCT image of an impacted tooth # 9 subsequent to such a mesiodens. Never before have we been able to determine such an exact position of these displaced and impacted central incisors. The position of these teeth and the root and crown morphology can be evaluated. This knowledge can help determine the desirability of retaining and placing traction on these impacted teeth. Many times, the orthodontist is the first to recognize the presence of supernumerary teeth or odontomas in the young patient. Two-dimensional radiographs, especially panoramic ones, can make definitive diagnosis of an early-forming supernumerary tooth difficult. The CBCT image allows a more exacting view to help determine the presence and position of these unwanted surprises.

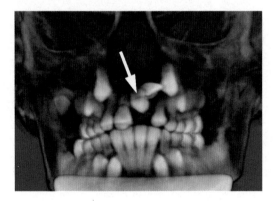

Fig. 2. CBCT image showing a mesiodens (*arrow*) that has deviated the maxillary left central incisor to a horizontal position.

Second molars can also become impacted and malpositioned, which can be caused by ectopically positioned adjacent third molars or second molar follicles that are inexplicably tipped in an oblique or horizontal orientation. If impinging third molars are not diagnosed and extracted appropriately, temporary or permanent delay in the eruptions of the second molars can be the result. Early diagnosis of these problems can lead to a significantly better prognosis of acceptable second molar eruption lending itself to orthodontic positioning on entry into the oral cavity. The author has found no other technique to compare with the diagnostic ability of the CBCT image in these situations. Fig. 3 shows a deviantly positioned third molar (#16) that was inhibiting proper eruption of tooth #15.

At times, the orthodontist desires to reposition the maxillary anterior teeth slightly in a first phase of treatment. On viewing the records, a mesiodens can be an unanticipated finding. If the oral surgeon wants to leave this mesiodens, and postpone its removal until a later date, the position of the mesiodens can be important. Delaying tooth movement must be considered if the mesiodens is in close proximity to the roots of the incisors. The orthodontist may pursue limited movement without significant fear of complications if the mesiodens in question is some distance from the roots. Using these images, the orthodontist and oral surgeon can combine their knowledge to establish a treatment plan that directs attention to the timing of mesiodens removal.

Root resorption

Most root resorption involved in orthodontic treatment can be readily viewed on periapical radiographs. However, resorption that occurs on the

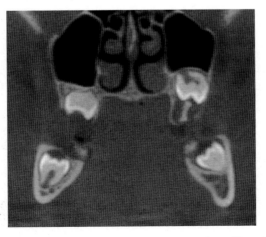

Fig. 3. Coronal CBCT image showing a deviantly positioned maxillary third molar (#16) inhibiting eruption of the second molar (#15).

814   HECHLER

facial or lingual side of the tooth is difficult to ascertain and quantify with
this 2D view. CBCT scanning allows for better viewing of resorption on
either of these surfaces [12]. However, the most important relationship of
CBCT imaging to root resorption may be that of determining maxillary
canine eruption position and its possible relationship with future spontane-
ous resorption of the adjacent lateral and central incisors. Removal of the
deciduous canine adjacent to the impacted permanent canine has been
shown to be effective if accomplished early [10]. Routine CBCT imaging
of the young patient for no apparent reason may be considered an inappropriate and excessive use of radiation. However, if one sees imminent danger
of resorption because of deviant canines on other films such as panoramic or
periapical radiographs, a follow-up CBCT image may be advisable.

Fractured roots

In the past, periapical radiographs have proved to be the best diagnostic
images for evaluating a patient for fractured roots. To view these fractures
radiographically may be difficult if the fracture is in an oblique direction and
not parallel to the beam of radiation supplying the radiograph image. Periapical radiographs can be difficult to take immediately post trauma because
of swelling, bleeding, and discomfort experienced by these patients. On the
contrary, CBCT scans can be acquired quickly and the teeth of interest may be
viewed from various angles and directions. The ability to view the cut of
a single tooth of interest in the three planes of space makes determining if
the involved tooth displays fracture much easier. The CBCT image of a young
man originally thought to have undergone fracture of only tooth #8 when
viewing the posttraumatic periapical radiograph is displayed in Fig. 4.
Further review of the CBCT image also indicated an oblique fracture of

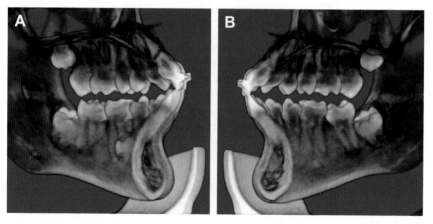

Fig. 4. (*A*) CBCT sagittal image displaying a horizontal root fracture of the maxillary right
central incisor (#8). (*B*) Image of #9 showing an oblique root fracture.

tooth #9. Not only the presence of root fracture but also the degree of displacement can be readily evaluated. Attempted movement of posttraumatic teeth with undiagnosed root fractures can greatly complicate the orthodontist's success in dealing with these cases. Moving the crowns while leaving the roots behind is never the desired outcome of orthodontic treatment.

Orthodontic temporary anchorage device placement

The temporary anchorage device (TAD) has gained popularity of late for use in orthodontic treatment. Many tooth movements that were mechanically difficult to accomplish in the past have become achievable with the use of these mini-implants. The placement of TADs by the orthodontist is becoming more common, although TADs will continue to be placed by the oral surgeon. In either case, the knowledge of the root positioning can greatly enhance the opportunity for proper placement and success of TADs [13]. CBCT images allow more accurate and dependable views of the interradicular relationships than panoramic radiographs [14]. These images allow not only more successful placement but also better treatment planning of where these TADs should be placed so that proper force vectors can be used during orthodontic treatment. CBCT data can be used to construct placement guides for positioning mini-implants between the roots of adjacent teeth in anatomically difficult sites [15].

The quality of the bone in the proposed placement sites can be evaluated before insertion of the mini-implants. Quantifying the thickness of the palatal bone can aid in determining the size and location of any TADs that may be treatment planned for the palate. CBCT images have been shown to be an accurate way to assess the volume of bone present at the proposed location [16]. The use of TADs will continue to increase in orthodontics, and retention of these mini-implants will be important to the successful outcome of treatment. The number of orthodontists using CBCT scans and TADs will increase significantly in the near future because these are common topics in the orthodontic literature and at seminars throughout the country.

Asymmetry evaluation

It can be difficult to evaluate the bony asymmetry of orthodontic patients using cephalometric and panoramic radiographs. Superimposition of structures, patient positioning, and distortion can be frustrating and unreliable. For instance, the comparison of the condyle and ramus lengths can be important to the occlusion of an orthodontic patient. Direct measurements can be made of these structures with CBCT imaging by comparing the right and left sides. Evaluation of mandibular asymmetry by way of CBCT imaging eliminates positioning problems. Imaging can provide measurements of mandibular anatomy either through 2D panoramic reconstructions or the entire 3D data package [17]. Software companies are adding the ability to extract (segment) the mandible or maxilla from the CBCT image and evaluate the bone independent of the other structures.

In addition, the unilateral nature of posterior crossbites can be diagnosed more specifically. The determination as to the presence of a truly unilateral crossbite versus one subsequent to a shift of the mandible into centric occlusion can be enhanced. A determination of an asymmetric maxilla or mandible can be accomplished more easily by viewing and measuring the bones in 3D. The orthodontist can view these structures in various angulations using the data taken in only one scan instead of using numerous 2D radiographic views.

Temporomandibular joint degenerative changes

Panoramic radiography is an acceptable initial tool for the assessment of temporomandibular joint (TMJ) osseous structures. But because of the known limitations of panoramic radiography, the absence of radiographic findings in a symptomatic patient does not rule out obscured osseous changes; moreover, radiographic findings, if present, may not be revealed in full.

Conventional tomography has been used extensively for the evaluation of TMJ hard tissues; however, technique sensitivity and the length of the examinations made it a less attractive diagnostic tool for the dental practitioner. CBCT images not only can be taken in the office but also viewed from many different angles and from an almost infinite number of slices. CBCT images of the TMJ have been shown to provide greater reliability and accuracy than tomographic or panoramic views in detecting condylar erosions [18]. With temporomandibular dysfunction continuing to be a haunting pathology in some orthodontic cases, it is important to view the anatomy of these patients' joints carefully before, during, and after orthodontic treatment. Follow-up CBCT images made over an extended period of time can be important to the orthodontist in evaluating the process of any degenerative changes that he or she may suspect. Current software solutions allow the visualization of TMJ osseous elements isolated (segmented) from other surrounding structures.

Cleft lip and palate

Estimates of the size (dimensions) of the osseous defects and the spatial relationship of the defect to other important anatomic structures are difficult to obtain in 2D images. CBCT can provide the cleft's exact anatomic relationships and bone thickness around the existing teeth in proximity to the cleft or clefts. This information is invaluable for the grafting procedures planned and for possible tooth movement in the existing dentition (Fig. 5).

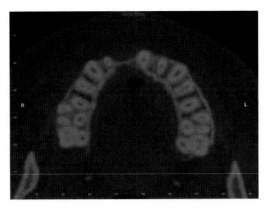

Fig. 5. Axial CBCT image of a patient who has a unilateral cleft and missing central incisor (#8).

Soft tissue

In the past, soft tissue evaluation was difficult using 2D photographs and radiographs. The patient's profile has been the most common soft tissue projection evaluated using photographs and lateral cephalometric radiographs. The profile is visualized using photographs; however, tracings and landmark analysis of the profile are quantified using the soft tissue observed on the lateral cephalometric radiograph. Although the profile is used by every orthodontist, many practitioners realize that patients seldom see their profile and are usually interested in the frontal view, which they are more apt to spend time viewing in the mirror. This view is also the one seen by others during day-to-day conversations.

Frontal photographs are used to judge symmetry, but without numerous views from different angles, it is difficult to gain a good feel of facial symmetry. Using the soft tissue data gathered in the CBCT scan, it is possible to rotate and tilt the head in an infinite number of positions to evaluate symmetry of the soft tissue. The positioning of the nose, the alar base fullness, and the inferior border of the mandible are only a few of the items easily studied. Surface area and volume analysis will surely be used in the future to aid in evaluating facial symmetry.

It is difficult to gain a good view of the nose with some CBCT machines because this area is at the edge of the image package. The author has found it much easier to gain good soft tissue imaging of the nose in younger individuals rather than in adults. The larger the nose, the less reliable the image can be. Recently, various companies have offered photographic imaging packages to coordinate with the CBCT data, using multiple camera locations. These systems are not widely used, but their use may increase as the cost decreases. Anatomage (Anatomage Inc., San Jose, California) currently has a process to take a common 2D digital facial photograph and map it to the CBCT image without the use of numerous cameras.

Airway

Using lateral cephalometric radiographs, the orthodontist may evaluate the airway in a 2D manner. Many studies have been accomplished and various analyses established in this way [19–21]. All this evaluation, however, is limited by the fact that we are looking at a flat projection seen in a sagittal or coronal plane. A 3D view of the airway can be readily available with CBCT imaging. Using CBCT images filtered to show airway, it is possible to quantify the volume of the airway and sinuses. The most constricted location of the airway can be found, and the axial view of this region can be quantified (Fig. 6). Orthodontists who are keenly interested in studying the patient's airway will surely continue to enhance the analyses that are available using the 3D information.

Future uses for cone-beam CT

Technology is constantly changing, and new applications arise almost daily. As of this writing, the following items give a glimpse of what may be available in the near future.

Virtual models

Plaster casts have been used in orthodontics for more than 100 years. They have been used to evaluate the patient's alignment, arch width, occlusion, tooth mass, and soft tissue. Smaller voxel size and innovative software have led to the ability to reconstruct virtual orthodontic study models

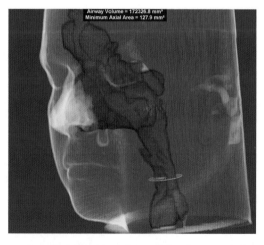

Fig. 6. CBCT airway view displaying the volume of the airway and sinuses. The most constricted region has been located and the minimum axial area calculated. (*Courtesy of* Dolphin Imaging and Management Solutions, Chatsworth, CA; with permission.)

without the need to obtain alginate impressions, which seems to be one of the most undesirable aspects of orthodontic treatment for our patients. CBCT data can be used to produce 3D models without the need for alginate impressions [22]. These virtual models can be composed with or without roots evident (Fig. 7). For many orthodontists, the presence of roots could be a major improvement over commonly used plaster casts, which only display the crowns. Also, these virtual models can be studied and measurements made on the computer, as is possible with those fabricated currently by the OrthoCad system (Cadent, Inc., Carlstadt, New Jersey) using impressions. If "hardcopy" models are needed, these can be fabricated from wax, starch, and plaster, using rapid prototyping technology [23].

Invisalign

The Invisalign (Align Technology, Santa Clara, California) tooth movement system was introduced to orthodontics in 1999. A series of clear thermoplastic trays are used to gain the desired tooth movement. These removable, computer-generated trays are changed every 2 weeks until the desired alignment and occlusion are gained. Currently, the orthodontist supplies the Invisalign laboratory polyvinyl siloxane impressions and a bite registration. The laboratory uses a computer linked to a destructive scanner to assemble this information into 3D renderings of the patient's teeth. These virtual models are adjusted on a computer per the orthodontist's detailed prescription of tooth movement. Once approved, the

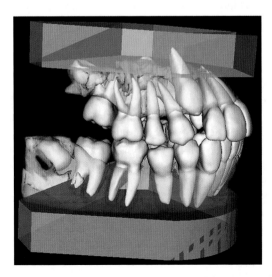

Fig. 7. Virtual models constructed from CBCT data without alginate impressions. (*Courtesy of* Anatomage Inc., San Jose, CA. Available at: http://www.anatomage.com. Accessed June 27, 2008; with permission.)

computer images are converted to "hardcopy" models using stereolithography and the clear trays are fabricated from these models [24].

It may be possible in the future to execute the entire fabrication process of the aligners using CBCT digital data. The CBCT images could be used to create the virtual models, thus negating the need to take and mail impressions and a bite registration. This information could be transferred electronically to certain laboratories (eg, Align Technologies), and the desired virtual tooth movement can be accomplished by way of e-mail communication between the orthodontist and the laboratory. Even the retainers could be fabricated by the data in the laboratory computer database of the final tooth positions.

Indirect bonding of brackets

Indirect bonding of fixed orthodontic brackets is used by many orthodontists to place these brackets on the teeth more accurately. Currently, in this technique, brackets are adhered to accurate stone models in the desired position. This bracket set-up is then transferred from the models to the patient using various types of trays and composite material. This laboratory fabrication is done either in the orthodontic office or at an outside facility. Construction of "hardcopy" models from the CBCT images could allow this indirect bonding to occur in either of these laboratory sites. If accomplished in an outside laboratory, the digital image could be electronically transferred to this laboratory with no pouring up or mailing of impressions involved. The same CBCT file used for the virtual models described earlier could be used for the indirect bonding procedure. Thus, patients could forgo two sets of the impressions they may dread.

Insignia

The Insignia process (Ormco Corporation, Orange, California) uses 3D imaging data and precision manufacturing to custom make orthodontic brackets and wires for an individual patient. Using an accurate impression taken by the orthodontist, the Insignia laboratory digitally constructs a virtual model of the teeth using specialized 3D scanners. Insignia software integrates these precision images with the orthodontist's prescription to calculate the optimum alignment and occlusion. The bracket for each tooth is then custom fabricated, taking into account the shape of the labial surface of the tooth and its root angulation and overall anatomy. An indirect bonding transfer mechanism is then fabricated so that each bracket may be placed at a specific location on each individual tooth. Wires are fabricated by the laboratory to work closely with the custom brackets to supply the desired orthodontic tooth movement.

It is anticipated that an accurate CBCT scan will replace the impression currently taken by the doctor. Ormco states that beta testing of the Insignia project in the clinical setting will begin sometime in 2008. Two of the biggest obstacles in taking such a leap (use of CBCT images for this type of fabrication) include patient motion and metallic artifacts (image deterioration due to presence of metal restorations), both of which may significantly affect the image quality, and thus the accuracy, of the virtual models that would be used during the Insignia process. According to the manufacturer, the available software would require the CBCT data to have been acquired with a voxel size between 0.05 and 0.07 mm, which is not offered yet by CBCT technologies.

Suresmile

Suresmile technology (OraMetrics, Inc., Richardson, Texas) uses the precision wire-bending capability of robots, combined with digital 3D scanning of teeth, computer simulation, and special wire materials to facilitate orthodontic tooth movement in an accurate fashion. This system uses a hand-held, 3D white-light scanning device to gain a virtual image of the patient's dentition. This procedure, done either through intraoral scanning or scanning of dental models, can be achieved with or without orthodontic brackets in place. These virtual images, along with the orthodontic prescription, are then used to position the dentition in its most aligned and interdigitated state. Wires are made by the Suresmile robot from a high-tech and flexible material to reposition the teeth orthodontically to the desired occlusion and alignment. Additional scans are usually taken during treatment to refine the tooth movement.

OraMetrics has been clinically beta testing the use of CBCT imaging to supply the virtual images of the teeth since the latter half of 2007. Voxel size of 0.2 mm or smaller is necessary to use this technology accurately. The accuracy of CBCT images in the Suresmile system again may be affected by patient motion and artifacts. Current software cannot adequately image all types of orthodontic brackets because of their composition. Plastic brackets seem to be the most difficult to visualize in CBCT scans. In the future, CBCT images could take the place of current orthodontic impressions and white-light scanning.

Summary

Orthodontists have used an arsenal of radiographs to diagnose and treatment plan their patients' cases carefully. Cephalometric, panoramic, periapical, and other radiographs have generally been 2D representations of 3D anatomic structures. CBCT offers a 3D image that can be used to aid in orthodontic tooth movement in all three planes of space. The use of CBCT data in the near future will change the way records are taken and treatment is rendered. Taking, pouring, or mailing impressions may become obsolete as the accuracy of CBCT scans improves. The computerization we have begun to rely on will take us to a level previously unimaginable.

Acknowledgments

The author thanks Mrs. Laura Gurwell for her invaluable help in typing and aiding in the organization of this article.

References

[1] Rakosi T. Cephalometry and radiographic analysis. In: Carruthers GB, editor. An atlas and manual of cephalometric radiography. London: Wolfe Medical Publications Ltd; 1982. p. 7.

[2] Moshiri M, Scarfe W, Hilgers M, et al. Accuracy of linear measurements from imaging plate and lateral cephalometric images derived from cone-beam computed tomography. Am J Orthod Dentofacial Orthop 2007;132(4):550–60.

[3] Langland O, Langlais R, McDavid W, et al. History of panoramic radiography. In: Panoramic radiography. 2nd edition. Philadelphia: Lea & Febiger; 1989. p. 3–37.

[4] Hutchison S. Cone beam computed tomography panoramic images versus traditional panoramic radiographs [thesis abstract]. Am J Orthod Dentofacial Orthop 2005;128(4):550.

[5] Elefteriadis J, Athanasiou A. Evaluation of impacted canines by means of computerized tomography. Int J Adult Orthodon Orthognath Surg 1996;11(3):257–64.

[6] Stewart J, Heo G, Glover K, et al. Factors that relate to treatment duration for patients with palatally impacted maxillary canines. Am J Orthod Dentofacial Orthop 2001;119(3):216–25.

[7] Walker L, Enciso R, Mah J. Three-dimensional localization of maxillary canines with cone-beam computed tomography. Am J Orthod Dentofacial Orthop 2005;128(4):418–23.

[8] Kokich V. Surgical and orthodontic management of impacted maxillary canines. Am J Orthod Dentofacial Orthop 2004;126(3):278–83.

[9] Ericson S, Kurol J. Resorption of maxillary lateral incisors caused by ectopic eruption of the canines. A clinical and radiographic analysis of predisposing factors. Am J Orthod Dentofacial Orthop 1988;94(6):503–13.

[10] Ericson S, Kurol J. Early treatment of palatally erupting maxillary canines by extraction of the primary canine. Eur J Orthod 1988;10(4):283–95.

[11] Kokich V, Mathews D. Impacted teeth: orthodontic and surgical considerations. In: McNamara J, Brudon W. Orthodontics and dentofacial orthopedics. 2nd edition. Ann Arbor (MI): Needham Press, Inc.; 2002. p. 395–422.

[12] Herring J. The effectiveness of orthodontists and oral radiologists in the diagnosis of impacted maxillary canines [thesis abstract]. Am J Orthod Dentofacial Orthop 2007; 132(6):861.

[13] Kuroda S, Yamada K, Deguchi T, et al. Root proximity is a major factor for screw failure in orthodontic anchorage. Am J Orthod Dentofacial Orthop 2007;131(4 Suppl):S68–73.

[14] Peck J, Sameshima G, Miller A, et al. Mesiodistal root angulation using panoramic and cone beam CT. Angle Orthod 2007;77(2):206–13.

[15] Kim S, Choi Y, Hwang E, et al. Surgical positioning of orthodontic mini-implants with guides fabricated on models replicated with cone-beam computed tomography. Am J Orthod Dentofacial Orthop 2007;131(4 Suppl):S82–9.

[16] King K, Lam E, Faulkner M, et al. Vertical bone volume in the paramedian palate of adolescents: a computed tomography study. Am J Orthod Dentofacial Orthop 2007; 132(6):783–8.

[17] Ludlow J, Laster W, See M, et al. Accuracy of measurements of mandibular anatomy in cone beam computed tomography images. Oral Surg Oral Med Oral Pathol Oral Radiol Endod 2007;103(4):534–42.

[18] Honey O, Scarfe W, Hilgers M, et al. Accuracy of the cone-beam computed tomography imaging of the temporomandibular joint: comparisons with panoramic radiology and linear tomography. Am J Orthod Dentofacial Orthop 2007;132(4):429–38.

[19] Compadretti G, Tasca I, Alessandri-Bonetti G, et al. Acoustic rhinometric measurements in children undergoing rapid maxillary expansion. Int J Pediatr Otorhinolaryngol 2006;70(1): 27–34.

[20] Battagel J, L'Estrange P. The cephalometric morphology of patients with obstructive sleep apnea. Eur J Orthod 1996;18(6):557–69.

[21] Athanasiou A, Papdopoulos M, Mazaheri M, et al. Cephalometric evaluation of pharynx, soft palate, adenoid tissue, tongue, and hyoid bone following the use of a mandibular repositioning appliance in obstructive sleep apnea patients. Int J Adult Orthodon Orthognath Surg 1994;9(4):273–83.

[22] Mah J. The evolution of digital study models. J Clin Orthod 2007;4(9):557–61.

[23] Macchi A, Carrafiello G, Cacciafesta V, et al. Three-dimensional digital modeling and set up. Am J Orthod Dentofacial Orthop 2006;129(5):605–10.

[24] Wong B. Invisalign A to Z. Am J Orthod Dentofacial Orthop 2002;121(5):540–1.

ELSEVIER
SAUNDERS

THE DENTAL
CLINICS
OF NORTH AMERICA

Dent Clin N Am 52 (2008) 825–841

Cone-Beam CT Diagnostic Applications: Caries, Periodontal Bone Assessment, and Endodontic Applications

Donald A. Tyndall, DDS, MSPH, PhD*,
Sonali Rathore, BDS

*Division of Oral and Maxillofacial Radiology, University of North Carolina
School of Dentistry, Brauer Hall, Chapel Hill, NC 27599-7450, USA*

In this issue of *Dental Clinics of North America*, cone-beam computed tomography (CBCT) applications in dentistry are examined. This article focuses on applications of CBCT to dentoalveolar disease and conditions, as applied in the practice of general dentistry, periodontics, and endodontics.

The technology of CBCT is described elsewhere in this issue of *Dental Clinics* and will not be repeated in detail here. It suffices to say that CBCT is a new application of CT that generates three-dimensional (3D) data at lower cost and absorbed doses than conventional CT found in the practice of medical radiology. Data from the craniofacial region are often collected at higher resolution in the axial plane than those from conventional CT systems [1]. In addition, these systems do not require a large amount of space and can easily fit into most dental practices today.

Most of the attention regarding CBCT imaging has focused on applications for dental implant placement, orthodontics, surgery, and temporomandibular joint imaging [2–8], and not as much emphasis has been placed on the applications of CBCT to dentoalveolar conditions and treatment. This article reviews and examines the available evidence from the clinical and scientific literature pertaining to dentoalveolar tasks, primarily limited to three basic areas: (1) caries diagnosis, (2), detection and characterization of the bony aspects of periodontal disease, and (3) endodontic applications, including the diagnosis of periapical lesions due to pulpal inflammation, visualization of canals, elucidation of internal and external resorption, and detection of root fractures.

---

* Corresponding author.
E-mail address: don_tyndall@dentistry.unc.edu (D.A. Tyndall).

0011-8532/08/$ - see front matter © 2008 Elsevier Inc. All rights reserved.
doi:10.1016/j.cden.2008.05.002
dental.theclinics.com

The chief limitation of current conventional intraoral and panoramic imaging for these common dentoalveolar diseases is the problem of conspicuity [9], which is largely the result of the representation of a 3D structure depicted by a two-dimensional (2D) image. This limitation is true for caries [10] and periodontal [11] and endodontic applications [9]. Dentistry has largely used the same method of 2D imaging since the first intraoral radiograph obtained in 1896. In fact, on close examination, only one or two significant advances in dental imaging have been made since then. These advances include panoramic imaging and tomography, with the former being far more useful for dental applications, and the latter historically being limited primarily to temporomandibular joint and implant site imaging. Digital imaging has been an advancement, yet the imaging geometry has not changed with these commonly used intraoral and panoramic technologies.

Earlier attempts have been made to improve the diagnosis and treatment of dentoalveolar conditions with 3D imaging using variations of tomosynthesis, most notably, tuned aperture CT (TACT) imaging [12]. Although TACT provided some incremental benefit for periodontal and endodontic applications, improvements in caries detection and characterization were limited to simulated recurrent caries [13–18]. These tomosynthetic methods proved promising but thus far have found limited application in the practice of dentistry. A new type of tomosynthetic technology, based on statistical inversion methods, named volume tomography, has recently entered the dental imaging market and may prove useful. It produces a stack of 256 images depicting cross-sectional information useful for implant treatment planning, which can visualize a limited volume of 6.0 by 6.0 cm. The system is an option with an OP 200 panoramic unit (Instrumentarium Dental, Tuusula, Finland) and is lower in cost and radiation dose than CBCT systems.

By the end of the twentieth century and the beginning of the twenty-first, it has become apparent that CBCT imaging may indeed be the next major advancement in dentoalveolar imaging, providing true 3D imaging at a lower cost than conventional CT, with radiation risks similar to current methods of intraoral imaging, including panoramic and full-mouth radiographic examination [19]. The advantages of CBCT for other maxillofacial applications have been well documented in this issue of *Dental Clinics*. What follows is a review of what is known about the potential benefits of CBCT imaging as applied to dentoalveolar tasks defined in this article as caries diagnosis, characterization of periodontal lesions, and various endodontic applications.

When considering a comparison of different imaging technologies, the reader is reminded that an increase in efficacy or lack thereof does not necessarily imply superiority or inferiority. Other factors must also be considered. A consideration of the total radiation risks for current imaging modalities, and ease of use and efficiency, should be considered. An example would be comparing CBCT with a full-mouth series of intraoral radiographs for the detection of dentoalveolar disease. CBCT would not necessarily have to demonstrate a superior diagnostic efficacy over a conventional full-mouth series of radiographs in order to be considered an improvement over conventional methods. If CBCT was equal to a full-mouth series in efficacy, it could be argued that, depending on machine type, the radiation risk would be considerably less, as would the time and effort it takes to image the patient. The reader may conclude that CBTC, under the aforementioned conditions, would actually be considered superior to conventional intraoral imaging methods. Alternative examinations such as a panoramic, with bitewings and limited periapical radiographs, might prove to have risks equal to, or fewer than, CBCT. In addition, the presence of metal effectively eliminates the possibility of caries detection in restored teeth, so CBCT may not prove practical for many patients as a general dental examination method unless it is supplemented with bitewing radiographs. Finally, in vitro studies involve no patient motion. Motion can, and often does, lead to CBCT image degradation. With these considerations in mind, the current literature on CBCT for caries diagnosis, periodontal bone characterization, and endodontic applications is examined, followed by a summary of what we know and can apply to current dental practice now and in the future.

Caries diagnosis

The detection of proximal and occlusal surface caries by conventional intraoral 2D methods has demonstrated only low-to-moderate sensitivity, but slightly better specificity, and high observer variability [20–26]. Pervious extraoral imaging methods for caries detection have met with limited success and dubious clinical applications. CBCT imaging appears to be the best prospect for improving the detection and depth assessment of caries in approximal and occlusal lesions. Recent work with benchtop-based local or limited CBCT (LCT) systems has demonstrated the potential for caries detection and depth characterization by high-resolution systems [10,27–30]. All five studies used a benchtop CBCT system with a high resolution (40-μm pixel) charge-coupled device (CCD) detector and rotating turntable with a fixed anode intraoral radiograph source; they also used histologically generated ground truth and small sample sizes of 24 to 30 teeth. LCT images were presented in parasagittal (similar to the bitewing view) and axial planes and were compared with bitewing radiographs. General linear model and receiver operating characteristic curves with analysis of variance methods were the statistical methods used. Kalathingal and colleagues [10] found no difference in the detection of carious lesions but did find that LCT was superior for caries depth assessment and although sensitivity increased, specificity showed no difference. The work performed by van Daatselaar and co-workers [27–30] demonstrated the superiority of LCT images for caries detection and noted that the number of source images could be as low as 14, a significant finding because a CCD detector was used for the study.

Turning to clinical CBCT systems, Akdeniz and coworkers [31] and Tsuchida and colleagues [32] used a limited-volume CBCT (LCBCT) Accuitomo device and compared in vitro CBCT results with either conventional film radiography or storage phosphor (SP) images. Akdeniz and colleagues, using 41 teeth, histologically verified ground truth, and all image planes for viewing found that LCBCT was superior for caries depth assessment when compared with SP and film. These results corroborated the work of Kalathingal and colleagues [10]. One possible weakness of the study was its use of only two observers.

Tsuchida and colleagues used micro-CT verified ground truth on 50 teeth with noncavitated incipient lesions, in a study where only 29 of the 100 surfaces were sound. Seven observers were used to generate receiver operating characteristic curves, which demonstrated no significant differences between the LCBCT images and film. This finding is not surprising, considering the difficulty of detecting incipient lesions.

A most recent and thorough study using full-volume CBCT and LCBCT by Haiter-Neto and colleagues [33] compared the NewTom 3G system (APF Imaging, Elmsford, New York) using three fields of view (12, 9, and 6 inches), the Accuitomo LCBCT system (J. Morita Manufacturing Corporation, Kyoto, Japan), Insight film (Eastman Kodak Company, Rochester, New York), and Digora SP (Soredex, Tuusula, Finland) images for the detection of approximal and carious lesions. Ground truth was histologically determined with 63% sound surfaces for approximal lesions and 6% for sound surfaces, with the former being the most realistic distribution of lesions to date which actually approximates interproximal caries prevalence. Six observers viewed all three fields of view for the NewTom system and all other modalities. The results showed that the NewTom 12-inch and 9-inch images had significantly lower sensitivities than the Accuitomo systems, whereas the NewTom 9-inch and 6-inch images had significantly lower specificities than the insight film and Digora images. The Accuitomo images were determined to be no different from film or the Digora-based images. For occlusal surfaces, the Accuitomo presented a higher sensitivity than the other systems. Specificity and overall true score did not differ among the modalities for occlusal lesions. The investigators concluded that the NewTom 3G system had a lower diagnostic accuracy for caries detection than the intraoral or LCBCT systems. The LCBCT systems were determined to be equal to the intraoral systems but did score higher in detecting dentinal lesions. These results are not surprising, given the lower spatial resolution of the NewTom system and the higher signal to noise ratio of the LCBCT system. Typically, the sensitivities were higher for the CBCT modalities but specificities were less, suggesting that one of the limitations of caries detection with CBCT imaging may be an increase in the number of false-positives. The investigators reminded the readers that CBCT doses for caries detection are still higher for many types of intraoral examinations, although they vary significantly, depending on which country is being studied. For instance, in the United

States, a full-mouth series of radiographs with D speed film and no rectangular collimation is the most common type of full-mouth radiographic examination. CCD-based, or even F speed with rectangular collimation, image series will be significantly less. Thus, the risks for CBCT imaging as a possible replacement for a full series of radiographs vary, depending on the system with which it is being compared.

The study did not separate the occlusal from the approximal lesions. Further studies are needed to evaluate CBCT for the detection of occlusal or pit and fissure caries, a task for which 2D imaging has been weak. In addition, the reader is reminded that in the in vitro studies mentioned earlier, intraoral 2D images were usually obtained under ideal geometry conditions with no closed contacts, cone cuts, or projective distortions. The equivalence of CBCT scores to those of 2D imaging may, in the minds of some, demonstrate the superiority of the former system. This point will also be considered in the conclusions. At this time, the application of CBCT imaging to caries diagnosis is promising, with more research needed, especially in vivo investigations. In addition, with current technology, it is assumed that teeth with metal or even radiopaque restorations should not be considered for CBCT caries imaging.

Examples of CBCT for caries imaging can be seen in Figs. 1 and 2.

Periodontal applications

In his 2004 summary of periodontal imaging methods in *Periodontology*, Mol states, "Relatively few technologies have emerged to address the critical needs in periodontal diagnosis" [11]. He goes on to point out that although digital imaging has added value to intraoral imaging, an increase in diagnostic capabilities has not been one of the benefits. Mol discusses the limitations of extraoral imaging (panoramic) with its associated drawbacks but does point

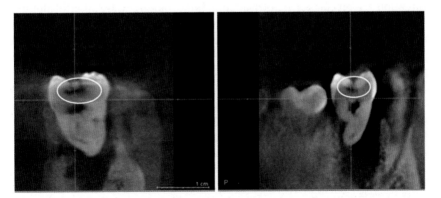

Fig. 1. Occlusal caries (*circled*) seen in a molar tooth from longitudinal and cross-sectional views. These images were part of an in vitro study using human teeth with histologically verified carious lesions. They were obtained using a 150-μm view with the Sirona Galileos CBCT system (Sirona Dental Systems, Bensheim, Germany).

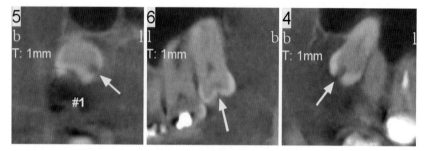

Fig. 2. Clinical caries seen in several molar teeth (*arrows*). These 300-μm images were obtained using the NewTom 3G system (APF Imaging Corp., Elmsford, New York).

out the usefulness in association with bitewings and selected periapicals. Mol also reviews the more advanced digital technologies, such as TACT, digital subtraction, and conventional CT scanning, and states their potential for an increase in diagnostic efficacy and characterization of the periodontal bone status. He concludes by outlining the practical limits of these technologies and explains why they are not going to be particularly useful in the practice of dentistry [11]. Previous studies have shown that CT assessment of alveolar bone height and bony pockets is reasonable, accurate, and precise [34–37]. Mol states that CBCT studies applied to periodontal imaging were in progress and not available at the time of publication of his review. Several of these studies are now available. Most studies investigating the application of CBCT imaging to periodontal bone status are in vitro, although a few are in vivo, with either full-volume CBCT or limited-volume units used.

Vandenberghe and coworkers [38] investigated periodontal bone architecture using 2D CCD and 3D full-volume CBCT-based imaging modalities. Periodontal bone levels and defects were assessed and evaluated against two human skulls' gold standard. Visualization of lamina dura, crater defects, furcation involvements, contrast, and bone quality were also evaluated. They concluded that CBCT image measurements of periodontal bone levels and defects were comparable to intraoral radiography. It was found that CBCT images demonstrated more potential in the morphologic description of periodontal bone defects and conversely, the CCD images provided more bone details. Using a dry skull with artificial defects and full-volume CBCT, Misch and colleagues [39] found similar results. Their investigation demonstrated that CBCT was as accurate as direct measurements using a periodontal probe and as reliable as radiographs for interproximal areas. In measurements of buccal and lingual defects, CBCT proved superior to conventional radiography. Because of this finding, the investigators concluded that CBCT offered a significant advantage over conventional radiography.

In a 2005 study using human and pig material, Mengel and coworkers [40] investigated the use of CBCT in the diagnosis of periodontal defects using intraoral radiography, panoramic radiography, CT, and LCBCT in comparison with histologic specimens. It was demonstrated that all intrabony defects could be measured in three planes in the CT and LCBCT scans with great accuracy true to scale, whereas only mesial, distal, and cranio-caudal plane defects could be detected by intraoral and panoramic imaging. It was also concluded that the LCBCT system produced higher-quality images. Noujeim and coworkers [41] found similar results when using the LCBCT system to detect simulated interradicular lesions of varying depth in comparison with intraoral radiography. Two studies in linear accuracy have recently been published by Loubele and colleagues and Mol and colleagues [42,43]. Loubele and coworkers designed a study to compare the accuracy of LCBCT with mul-tislice CT for linear measurements with caliper-determined measurements us-ing cadaveric materials. They concluded that both systems were accurate with submillimeter measures. In a study directed more to periodontal defects, Mol, using an older form of CBCT using a full field of view, found that CBCT im-ages provided better diagnostic and quantitative information on periodontal bone levels in three dimensions than conventional radiography. The study also demonstrated a limitation in that the accuracy in the anterior aspect of the jaws was limited. The system used a NewTom 9000 unit (APF Imaging, Elmsford, New York), generating images that were inferior in quality to what more up-to-date systems can generate.

The fact that these studies used full-volume CBCT and limited-volume systems hints that either system may be more capable than intraoral radiog-raphy in the visualization of periodontal bone architecture. The reader is reminded that motion can cause image degradation and that all the studies mentioned are in vitro and are not subject to the less than ideal clinical situation [44]. At the same time, intraoral radiography is featured in ideal conditions in these in vitro studies.

In a recent review of currently published literature on CBCT for peri-odontology, Kasaj and Willershausen [45] conclude that the low dosage and superior image quality in comparison with conventional CT are prom-ising for periodontal applications, especially in the areas of intrabony defects, dehiscence and fenestration defects, and periodontal cysts, and in the diagnosis of furcation-involved molars. This summary encapsulates the findings of the studies discussed earlier. Overall, these studies suggest that CBCT imaging has the potential to replace intraoral imaging for the assessment of periodontal architecture. However, clinical studies would be helpful in supporting this conclusion. CBCT may be a useful and more prac-tical clinical tool than digital subtraction radiography for the assessment of changes in periodontal bone over time. Examples of CBCT for periodontal imaging can be seen in Figs. 3 and 4.

Endodontic applications

It is in the area of endodontic applications that the literature has proved most fruitful to date. Endodontic applications include the diagnosis of peri-apical lesions due to pulpal inflammation, visualization of canals,

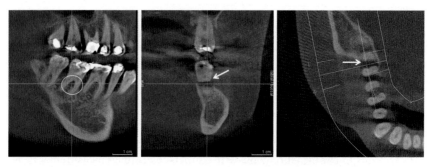

Fig. 3. Three images depicting a complete periodontal furcation involvement of a second molar. The figure on the left visualizes a furcation involvement delineated by the circle. The center and right images demonstrate the extent of the lesion (*arrows*) from facial-lingual and axial views. These 300-µm images were obtained with the Sirona Galileos CBCT system (Sirona Dental Systems, Bensheim, Germany).

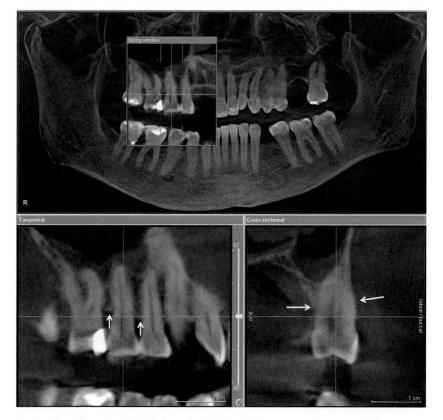

Fig. 4. Three-dimensional depiction of periodontal bone loss around a maxillary second premolar tooth. The arrows indicate the extent of bone loss on the facial, palatal, mesial, and distal aspects of the tooth. These 300-µm images were obtained with the Sirona Galileos CBCT system (Sirona Dental Systems, Bensheim, Germany).

elucidation of internal and external resorption, and detection of root fractures. As is the case with the previous two categories, most published articles are either case reports or in vitro studies.

Current 2D technologies are film and digital based. Stavropoulos and Wenzel [46] remarked in a recent article that the two have few, if any, differences. The investigators do point out that digital enhancements may result in limited improvement in detection. The classic study by Bender and Seltzer [47,48] demonstrated the limitations of intraoral radiography for the detection of periapical lesions. Their study revealed that in order for a lesion to be visible radiographically, the cortical plate of bone must be engaged. Many subsequent studies since that time have underscored the difficulty of detecting periapical lesions. These radiographic limitations are summarized in a review by Huumonen and Ørstavik [49], in which they state that such limitations exist, in part, because radiographs are 2D in nature and clinical or biologic features may not be reflected in radiographic changes.

Evidence is compelling that these limitations may be overcome through CBCT imaging. It is reviewed below.

A review of digital and 3D applications for endodontic uses recently published by Nair and Nair [50] summarized the CBCT portion by stating that such technology has proved useful for localization and characterization of root canals, treatment planning of periapical surgery, and detection of root fractures in extracted teeth. This last topic was explored in a recent in vitro study by Mora and coworkers [51], who used a benchtop high-resolution LCBCT device to demonstrate the superiority of this technology over conventional 2D imaging. Basis image sets of 180, 60, 32, and 20 were used and all but the 20 image group proved more accurate. The investigators point out that this study used a high-resolution CCD detector currently not used by any existing CBCT system.

In a clinical study conducted by Simon and coworkers [52], CBCT was found to be useful in differentiating solid from fluid-filled lesions (periapical granulomas from cysts) using grayscale values in the lesions. This information would presumably enable the clinician to manage the lesion in question more effectively. This study was one of the few that was clinical in nature and verified by histologic analysis. Of the total 17 lesions, 13 were correctly identified by CBCT. Of the remaining lesions, the investigators felt that the CBCT results were actually more accurate than the microscopic analysis because of poor biopsy sampling. Another clinically based publication, by Cotton and coworkers [53], featured a series of case reports demonstrating the usefulness of high-resolution LCBCT of endodontic applications. Such applications included identifying an untreated canal that had resulted in root canal treatment (RCT) failure, identifying a nondisplaced root fracture, identifying the extent of internal resorptions not seen on periapical radiographs, visualizing extruded RCT material in the mental nerve canal, and a few other applications. In all cases, the 3D nature of the CBCT images revealed aspects of a periapical or tooth area that had a positive influence on the clinical outcome. Although this study was not scientifically controlled, it did point to the various potential uses of CBCT for endodontic diagnosis and applications. A recent case report by Maini and coworkers [54] demonstrated the benefit of CBCT in identifying resorption of a tooth contacted by an impacted canine. In this case, orthodontics was not used and an alternative treatment plan was generated. In their article, the investigators pointed out that CBCT studies have shown that 68% of impacted canines cause root resorption of adjacent teeth, up from 12%, as determined from previous 2D studies [55].

Further clinical applications were demonstrated by Rigolone and coworkers [56] in a clinical study using large-volume CBCT as an aid in apicoectomy surgery involving the palatal root of a maxillary molar. In this clinical study based on 31 patients, CBCT was effective in identifying an alternative and less invasive surgical approach using a vestibular, as opposed to a palatal, approach in combination with an operating microscope. Tsurumachi and Honda [57] described the use of LCBCT in localizing a broken endodontic instrument in the maxillary sinus in yet another application for endodontic practice.

Patel and coworkers [58] reviewed the literature on CBCT applications to endodontics and found CBCT to be clinically superior to periapical radiography for the detection of periapical lesions. They cited an interesting study by Lofthag-Hansen and coworkers [59], in which CBCT was found to result in 62% more periapical lesions on individual roots being identified, when compared with periapical examinations. In addition, Patel and colleagues found CBCT to be efficacious in endodontic surgery, periapical surgery treatment planning, identification of root canals not seen on 2D images, identification of dentoalveolar trauma, and the management of external cervical root resorption. Furthermore, the investigators posit that one of the most important applications of CBCT imaging for endodontics may be in the assessment of treatment outcomes. They argue that the greater geometric accuracy of CBCT scans should prove superior to conventional imaging of treatment follow-through and the assessment of healing post-RCT.

Several important in vitro studies have been conducted that apply CBCT imaging to other endodontic applications [46,60]. In 2007, Sogur and colleagues [60] conducted a study comparing the subjective image quality of root canal fillings among LCBCT, SP, and film radiography. In that study, CBCT was found to be inferior to 2D digital radiographs because of the limitations of streaking artifacts. Finally, in the previously cited ex vivo investigation by Stavropoulos and Wenzel, a large-format CBCT system was compared with 2D digital and film images for the detection of simulated periapical lesions in pig jaws. In that study, cylindric defects of 1 mm × 1 mm, 2 mm × 2 mm, and 3 mm × 3 mm were randomly prepared beyond the apices of extraction sockets. Control sites were also included. Blinded examiners were used. CBCT images proved statistically superior in sensitivity,

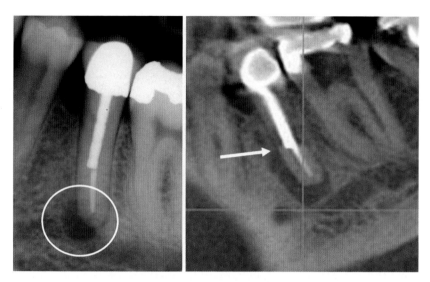

Fig. 5. In this case, the standard 2D periapical radiograph did not reveal the true extent of the apical lesion (*circle*). The pattern of the lesion suggests a root fracture (*arrow*). In this case, the treatment of the tooth was changed from re-treating the root canal to extracting the tooth. These 300-μm images were obtained with the Sirona Galileos CBCT system (Sirona Dental Systems, Bensheim, Germany).

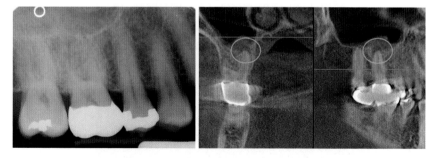

Fig. 6. In this case, a patient had a 3- to 4-month history of intermittent pain associated with a recently placed crown restoration. Multiple periapical radiographs were obtained but showed no evidence of a periapical lesion. The most recent periapical radiograph is shown on the left. The center and right figures are CBCT images that clearly depict a periapical lesion extending into the maxillary sinus. The circled areas indicate the lesion. Note also that most of the facial cortical plate of bone is preserved, possibly explaining why the lesion failed to appear on the periapical radiographs. These 300-μm images were obtained with the Sirona Galileos CBCT system (Sirona Dental Systems, Bensheim, Germany).

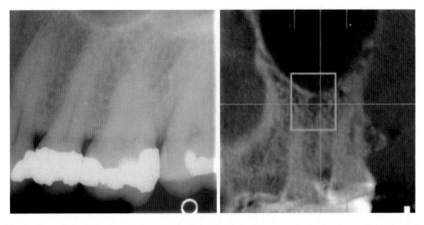

Fig. 7. In a case similar to Fig. 6, this patient had intermittent pain and returned to the clinic for repeated periapical radiographs, all of which were negative, as seen in the image on the left. The right image depicts the CBCT view of a small but definitive periapical lesion. In both cases, RCTs solved the patient's tooth-related problems. Figs. 6 and 7 are good examples of the limited diagnostic benefits of high-resolution 2D images. Despite having a lower resolution, the CBCT images were superior to the periapical radiographs for diagnosing the problems. These 300-μm images were obtained with the Sirona Galileos CBCT system (Sirona Dental Systems, Bensheim, Germany).

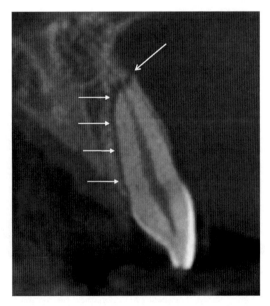

Fig. 8. This patient was struck in the mouth and suffered a facial cortical plate fracture (*open arrow*). This image demonstrates the usefulness of CBCT in assessing dentoalveolar trauma. In addition, a widened periodontal ligament space is visualized (*closed arrows*) on the lingual aspect, which most likely represents subluxation of the tooth. This 300-μm image was obtained with the Sirona Galileos CBCT system (Sirona Dental Systems, Bensheim, Germany).

positive and negative predictive values, and diagnostic accuracy when compared with the 2D modalities. Specificity was similar for all three methods.

In summary, in vivo and in vitro investigations demonstrate the superiority of CBTC to conventional imaging for almost all endodontic applications, except for assessing the quality of root canal fills. Although most studies were in vitro and were observational in nature, the usefulness of CBCT over 2D imaging was demonstrated. Of course, dose and costs must come into consideration when deciding the most appropriate selection criteria for CBCT imaging. Here, as in the other dentoalveolar applications, the reader is reminded that no double blind clinical trials or studies with other, more robust, in vivo research methodologies have taken place. However, such studies are time consuming and expensive and generally use technologies that are out of date by the time of publication; hence, the profession is left with less than ideal studies on which to base selection criteria decisions. The in vitro evidence is compelling but, again, the reader is reminded that these studies have no motion, which is perhaps balanced by the fact that 2D studies are undertaken with ideal imaging geometries that are seldom achieved in the clinic. Examples of CBCT for endodontic applications can be seen in Figs. 5 to 8.

Summary

In summary, several important points should be considered:

1. Only a modest amount of research has been undertaken in the field of CBCT and dentoalveolar applications. Certainly, more in vivo and in vitro studies are needed for this field to reach full maturation. More clinical studies are needed, preferably random double blind clinical trials. In addition, the effect of motion needs to be assessed for all three categories of dentoalveolar tasks surveyed in this article.
2. CBCT and caries research results are mixed for proximal caries and few data exist for occlusal and pit and fissure caries at this time.
3. CBCT imaging for caries should be limited to nonrestored teeth. Even so, we still do not know the effect of beam hardening on producing possible artifacts and false-positives. Apparently, sensitivity may increase with CBCT but it should not be at the cost of specificity.
4. As for periodontal disease, CBCT promises to be superior to 2D imaging for the visualization of bone topography and lesion architecture but no more accurate than 2D for bone height. This factor should be tempered with an awareness that restoration in the dentition may obscure views of the alveolar crest.
5. CBCT for endodontic purposes appears to be the most promising use of CBCT, in many instances instead of 2D images. Applications would include apical lesions, root fractures, canal identification, and characterization of internal and external root resorption.

Evidence is strong that CBCT imaging potentially could replace 2D intraoral imaging for most dentoalveolar tasks, especially in endodontic and periodontal applications. This possibility is especially worthy of consideration because mere diagnostic equivalency of CBCT and 2D systems may favor the former because imaging is faster and accompanied by fewer problems of geometric distortion. When considering such a shift in imaging strategy, dose and costs must come into consideration, balanced with the perspective that most CBCT studies are easier to perform in a dental office when compared with a full-mouth series of radiographs, or perhaps even a panoramic radiograph with bitewings and selected periapical images. In the United States, the radiation risks from many CBCT systems would be below those for the most common intraoral full-mouth series examination [19], which suggests that it may be possible, with the appropriate use of CBCT technology and selected intraoral images, to gain more information about dentoalveolar conditions and treatment with fewer risks and time, benefiting both the patient and the dentist. These postulates assume an increase in the availability of CBCT systems and a reasonable speed with which the dental profession adopts the technology. No doubt, future improvements in CBCT technology will result in systems with even more favorable diagnostic yields and lower doses. If a drop in prices occurs, then an age where CBCT imaging is the primary form of dental imaging may dawn. For now, CBCT imaging, like its medical counterpart, can be seen as a highly useful and, with some tasks, indispensable part of the dental imaging armamentarium.

References

[1] Ito K, Gomi Y, Sato S, et al. Clinical application of a new compact CT-system to assess 3-D images for the preoperative treatment planning of implants in the posterior mandible. A case report. Clin Oral Implants Res 2001;12:539–42.
[2] Lascala CA, Panella J, Marques MM. Analysis of the accuracy of linear measurements obtained by cone beam computed tomography (CBCT-NewTom). Dentomaxillofac Radiol 2004;33:291–4.
[3] Honda K, Arai Y, Kashima M, et al. Evaluation of the usefulness of the limited cone-beam CT (3DX) in the assessment of the thickness of the roof of the glenoid fossa of the temporomandibular joint. Dentomaxillofac Radiol 2004;33:391–5.
[4] Ziegler CM, Woertche R, Briefand J, et al. Clinical indications for digital volume tomography in oral and maxillofacial surgery. Dentomaxillofac Radiol 2002;31:126–30.
[5] Mozzo P, Procacci C, Tacconi A, et al. A new volumetric CT machine for dental imaging based on the conebeam technique: preliminary results. Eur Radiol 1998;8:1558–64.
[6] Danforth RA. Cone beam volume tomography: a new digital imaging option for dentistry. J Calif Dent Assoc 2003;31:814–5.
[7] Sukovic P. Cone beam computed tomography in craniofacial imaging. Orthod Craniofac Res 2003;6(Suppl 1):31–6.
[8] Scarfe CS. Imaging of maxillofacial trauma: evolutions and emerging revolutions. Oral Surg Oral Med Oral Pathol Oral Radiol Endod 2005;100:575–96.
[9] Kundel HL, Revesz G. Lesion conspicuity, structured noise, and film reader error. Am J Roentgenol 1976;126:1233–8.

[10] Kalathingal SM, Mol A, Tyndall DA, et al. In vitro assessment of cone beam local computed tomography for proximal caries detection. Oral Surg Oral Med Oral Pathol Oral Radiol Endod 2007;104:699–704.

[11] Mol A. Imaging methods in periodontology. Periodontol 2000;2004(34):34–8.

[12] Webber RL, Horton RA, Tyndall DA, et al. Tuned-aperture computed tomography (TACT): theory and application for 3-D dentoalveolar imaging. Dentomaxillofac Radiol 1997;26:53–62.

[13] Tyndall DA, Clifton LT, Webber RL, et al. TACT imaging of primary caries. Oral Surg Oral Med Oral Pathol Oral Radiol Endod 1997;84:214–25.

[14] Nair MK, Tyndall DA, Ludlow JB, et al. The effects of restorative material and lesion location on recurrent caries detection for Ektaspeed Plus film; direct digital radiography, and tuned aperture computed tomography (TACT). Dentomaxillofac Radiol 1998;27:80–4.

[15] Abreu M, Tyndall DA, Platin E, et al. Two- and three-dimensional imaging modalities for the detection of caries. A comparison between film, digital radiography and tuned aperture computed tomography. Dentomaxillofac Radiol 1999;28(3):152–7.

[16] Nance RS, Tyndall DA, Levin LG, et al. Diagnosis of external root resorption using TACT (tuned aperture computed tomography). Endodont and Trauma 2000;16(1):24–8.

[17] Nance RS, Tyndall DA, Levin LG, et al. Identification of root canals in molars by tuned-aperture computed tomography. Int Endod J 2000;33(4):392–6.

[18] Ramesh A, Ludlow JB, Webber RL, et al. Evaluation of tuned aperture computed tomography (TACT) in the localization of simulated periodontal defects. Dentomaxillofac Radiol 2001;30(6):319–24.

[19] Ludlow JB, Davies-Ludlow LE, Brooks SL, et al. Dosimetry of 3 CBCT devices for oral and maxillofacial radiology: CB Mercuray, NewTom 3G and I-Cat. Dentomaxillofac Radiol 2006;35:219–26.

[20] Hintze H, Christoffersen L, Wenzel A. In vitro comparison of Kodak ultra-speed, Ektaspeed, and Ektaspeed plus, and Agfa M2 comfort dental x-ray films for the detection of caries. Oral Surg Oral Med Oral Pathol Oral Radiol Endod 1996;81:240–4.

[21] Hintze H, Wenzel A, Danielsen B, et al. Reliability of visual examination, fibre-optic trans-illumination, and bitewing radiography, and reproducibility of direct visual examination following tooth separation for the identification of cavitated carious lesions in contacting approximal surfaces. Caries Res 1998;32:204–9.

[22] Hintze H, Wenzel A, Jones C. In vitro comparison of D- and E-speed film radiography, RVG, and Visualix digital radiography for the detection of enamel approximal and dentinal occlusal caries lesions. Caries Res 1994;28:363–7.

[23] Wenzel A, Borg E, Hintze H, et al. Accuracy of caries diagnosis in digital images from charge-coupled device and storage phosphor systems: an in vitro study. Dentomaxillofac Radiol 1995;24:250–4.

[24] White SC, Yoon DC. Comparative performance of digital and conventional images for detecting proximal surface caries. Dentomaxillofac Radiol 1997;26:32–8.

[25] Clifton TL, Tyndall DA, Ludlow JB. Alternative extraoral radiographic imaging of primary caries. Dentomaxillofac Radiol 1998;27:193–8.

[26] Khan E, Tyndall D, Caplan D, et al. Extra-oral imaging for proximal caries detection; bite-wings vs. scanogram. Oral Surg Oral Med Oral Pathol Oral Radiol Endod 2004;98(6):730–7.

[27] van Daatselaar AN, Dunn SM, Spoelder HJ, et al. Feasibility of local CT of dental tissues. Dentomaxillofac Radiol 2003;32:173–80.

[28] van Daatselaar AN, Tyndall DA, van der Stelt PF. Detection of caries with local CT. Dentomaxillofac Radiol 2003;32:235–41.

[29] van Daatselaar AN, Tyndall DA, Verheij H, et al. Minimum number of basis projections for caries detection with local CT. Dentomaxillofac Radiol 2004;33:355–60.

[30] van Daatselaar AN, van der Stelt PF, Weenen J. Effect of number of projections on image quality of local CT. Dentomaxillofac Radiol 2004;33:361–9.

[31] Akdeniz BG, Gröndahl HG, Magnusson B. Accuracy of proximal caries depth measurements: comparison between limited cone-beam CT, storage phosphor and film radiography.
Caries Res 2006;40:202–7.

[32] Tsuchida R, Araki K, Tomohiro Okano T. Evaluation of limited cone-beam volumetric
imaging system: comparison with film radiography in detecting incipient proximal caries.
Oral Surg Oral Med Oral Pathol Oral Radiol Endod 2007;104:412–6.

[33] Haiter-Neto F, Wenzel A, Gotfredsen E. Diagnostic accuracy of cone beam computed
tomography scans compared with intraoral image modalities for detection of caries lesions.
Dentomaxillofac Radiol 2008;37:18–22.

[34] Fuhrmann RAW, Bücker A, Diedrich PR. Assessment of alveolar bone loss with high
resolution computed tomography. J Periodont Res 1995;30:258–63.

[35] Fuhrmann RA, Wehrbein H, Langen HJ, et al. Assessment of the dentate alveolar process
with high resolution computed tomography. Dentomaxillofac Radiol 1995;24:50–4.

[36] Naito T, Hosokawa R, Yokota M. Three-dimensional alveolar bone morphology analysis
using computed tomography. J Periodontol 1998;69:584–9.

[37] Pistorius A, Patrosio C, Willershausen B, et al. Periodontal probing in comparison by CT-
scan. Int Dent J 2001;51:339–47.

[38] Vandenberghe B, Jacobs R, Yang J. Diagnostic validity (or acuity) of 2D CCD versus 3D
CBCT-images for assessing periodontal breakdown. Oral Surg Oral Med Oral Pathol
Oral Radiol Endod 2007;104:395–401.

[39] Misch KA, Yi ES, Sarment DP. Accuracy of cone beam computed tomography for periodontal defect measurements. J Periodontol 2006;77:1261–6.

[40] Mengel R, Candir M, Shiratori K, et al. Digital volume tomography in the diagnosis of periodontal defects: an in vitro study on native pig and human mandibles. J Periodontol 2005;
76(5):665–73.

[41] Noujeim M, Nummikoski P, Langlais R. Evaluation of high-resolution cone-beam computed tomography in the detection of simulated interradicular bone lesions. Oral Surg
Oral Med Oral Pathol Oral Radiol Endod 2007;103:e52.

[42] Loubele M, van Assche N, Carpentier K, et al. Comparative localized linear accuracy of
small-field cone-beam CT and multislice CT for alveolar bone measurements. Oral Surg
Oral Med Oral Pathol Oral Radiol Endod 2008;105:512–8.

[43] Mol A, Balasundaram A. In vitro cone beam computed tomography imaging of periodontal
bone. Dentomaxillofac Radiol 2008;37:1–6.

[44] Scarfe WC, Farman AG, Sukovis P. Clinical applications of cone-beam computed tomography in dental practice. J Can Dent Assoc 2006;72:75–80.

[45] Kasaj A, Willershausen B. Digital volume tomography for diagnostics in periodontology.
Int J Comput Dent 2007;10(2):155–68.

[46] Stavropoulos A, Wenzel A. Accuracy of cone beam dental CT, intra oral digital and conventional film radiography for the detection of periapical lesions. An ex vivo study in pig jaws.
Clin Oral Investig 2007;1:101–6.

[47] Bender B, Seltzer S. Roentgenographic and direct observation of experimental lesions in
bone I. J Am Dent Assoc 1961;62:152–60.

[48] Bender B, Seltzer S. Roentgenographic and direct observation of experimental lesions in
bone II. J Am Dent Ass 1961;62:708–16.

[49] Huumonen S, Ørstavik D. Radiological aspects of apical periodontitis. Endodontic Topics
2002;1:3–25.

[50] Nair M, Nair U. Digital and advanced imaging in endodontics: a review. J Endod 2007;33(1):
1–6.

[51] Mora MA, Mol A, Tyndall DA, et al. In vitro assessment of local computed tomography for
the detection of longitudinal tooth fractures. Oral Surg Oral Med Oral Pathol Oral Radiol
Endod 2007;103:825–9.

[52] Simon J, Reyes E, Malfaz J-M, et al. Differential diagnosis of large periapical lesions using
cone-beam computed tomography measurements and biopsy. J Endod 2006;32:833–7.

[53] Cotton TP, Geilser MG, Holden DT, et al. Endodontic applications of cone-beam volumetric tomography. J Endod 2007;33:1121–32.
[54] Maini A, Durning P, Drage N. Resorption: within or without? The benefit of cone-beam computed tomography when diagnosing a case of an internal/external resorption defect. Braz Dent J 2008;204:135–7.
[55] Walker L, Enciso R, Mah J. Three-dimensional localization of maxillary canines with cone-beam computed tomography. Am J Orthod Dentofacial Orthop 2005;128:418–23.
[56] Rigolone M, Pasqualini D, Bianchi L, et al. Vestibular surgical access to the palatine root of the superior first molar: "low-dose cone-beam" CT analysis of the pathway and its anatomic variations. J Endod 2003;29:773–5.
[57] Tsurumachi T, Honda K. A new cone beam computerized tomography system for use in endodontic surgery. Int Endod J 2007;40:224–32.
[58] Patel S, Dawood A, Pitt Ford T, et al. The potential applications of cone beam computed tomography in the management of endodontic problems. Int Endod J 2007;40:818–30.
[59] Lofthag-Hansen S, Huumonen S, Grö ndahl K, et al. Limited cone-beam CT and intraoral radiography for the diagnosis of periapical pathology. Oral Surg Oral Med Oral Pathol Oral Radiol Endod 2007;103:114–9.
[60] Sogur E, Baks BG, Grö ndahl H-G. Imaging of root canal fillings: a comparison of subjective image quality between limited conebeam CT, storage phosphor and film radiography. Int Endod J 2007;40:179–85.

THE DENTAL CLINICS
OF NORTH AMERICA

ELSEVIER
SAUNDERS

Dent Clin N Am 52 (2008) 843–873

Oral and Maxillofacial Pathology in Three Dimensions

Steven A. Guttenberg, DDS, MD[a,b,c,d,*]

[a]*Washington Institute for Mouth, Face and Jaw Surgery, 2021 K Street, NW,
Suite 200, Washington, DC 20006-1003, USA*
[b]*Department of Oral and Maxillofacial Surgery, Washington Hospital Center,
Washington, DC, USA*
[c]*Nova Southeastern University College of Dental Medicine, Fort Lauderdale, FL, USA*
[d]*Temple University, Philadelphia, PA, USA*

When pathologic lesions of the jaws are evaluated, a certain amount of information is gathered that is then distilled into the fabrication of a presumptive diagnosis, before surgical intervention (if that is necessary). Demographic information (age, sex, and race) is harvested. Patients are asked if they have certain complaints (pain, altered sensation, or anesthesia), or not. The facial structures are clinically examined for discolorations, depressions, swellings, and asymmetries. Laboratory studies may be indicated and ordered. And then, radiographic tools are used to evaluate that which we cannot see beneath the skin. The exposed images are examined, looking for the lesion's exact location (maxilla, mandible, anterior, posterior, alveolar process, and so forth). The exact size of the defect and its relative density (radiolucent or radiopaque or a combination) are determined.

Information about potential aggressiveness is sought. Does the lesion expand the cortex? Does it thin it or perforate it? Is it unilocular or multilocular? Is it unifocal or multifocal? What are the characteristics of the border? Is it smooth, ragged, or can one even discern a border. Are teeth involved? Are they impacted or have they been displaced? Have the roots been resorbed? To perfect an accurate diagnosis, these are the questions that must be answered. This will be facilitated by gathering as much information as possible. In general, the greater its quality, the better will be the diagnosis.

* Washington Institute for Mouth, Face and Jaw Surgery, 2021 K Street, NW, Suite 200, Washington, DC 20006-1003.
E-mail address: sag@mouthfacejaw.com

Plain film radiography

During the past 4 decades, dentistry has seen a dramatic expansion and refinement of the technology used to identify dental and intraosseous disorders. Whereas the profession had always depended on intraoral radiographs (primarily periapical bite wings and occlusals), during the 1960s, commercially available extraoral panoramic radiography became available for use in the dental office. This introduction allowed the practitioner to gain much more information about the teeth and jaws, especially if surgical intervention was being contemplated. During the next 40 years, the main advances were seen in improvement of film stock and techniques to shorten the time of exposure and thereby the absorbed dose of irradiation. The current advanced state of intraoral and panoramic radiography is highlighted by the replacement of film-based image capture by digital imaging.

During this time frame (and previously as well), when there was a need for more information, patients had to be sent to private or hospital-based medical radiology centers so that more major extraoral facial or skull x-rays could be taken. Examples of films that were routinely ordered are posteroanterior and oblique skull and jaws views, Townes and reverse Townes views, submentovertex and specific exposures of the paranasal sinuses, and tomograms.

With the introduction of tomography, diagnosticians were given an additional tool to evaluate lesions, the ability to look at an object in three dimensions. These films had an advantage over panoramic x-rays since distortion was not as prevalent as is seen in the latter. However, similar to panoramic radiography, the problem of image magnification persisted.

Digital radiography

Then in the 1980s computed tomograms (CTs) became available and many of the films that had been previously taken for evaluation of the facial skeleton began to fade from use. There is little question that at this point, CT is the standard for maxillofacial hard tissue evaluation. However, within the dental community, with the exception of major pathology or trauma, there was a hesitancy to use this technology. This was understandable because (1) patients had to be sent out of the office to have the studies performed; (2) there were large doses of irradiation for the patient; (3) the medical radiologist did not always appreciate the information that the dental practitioner was seeking; (4) there was a variable lag time between the patient being sent and the practitioner receiving the information; and (5) the scans were expensive. In addition, most dentists did not have the training or experience necessary to read and properly evaluate the radiographic work product that they received.

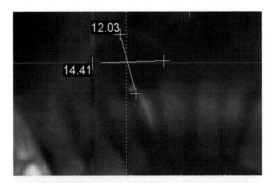

Fig. 1. Case 1. Detail from panoramic view revealing a 1.2 × 1.4 cm periapical radiolucency associated with the apex of the maxillary right lateral incisor tooth.

This changed at the beginning of the current century when the first cone beam computed tomography (CBCT) machines for dental office use became commercially available. These machines have created a new paradigm for the evaluation of dental and maxillofacial structures in the ambulatory setting. The units are much smaller than the medical CTs, are less expensive to purchase and operate, produce a fraction of the radiation dose, and possess an open architecture that, generally, eliminates patient complaints of claustrophobia.

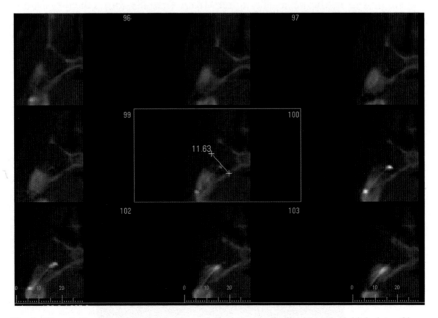

Fig. 2. Case 1. Cross-sectional views through the lesion indicating that the labial plate of bone has been destroyed. The nasal floor and palatal cortex are intact.

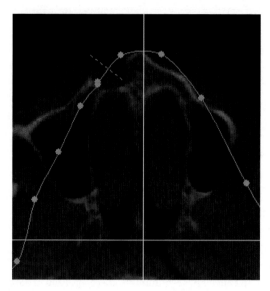

Fig. 3. Case 1. Axial view demonstrating the relationship of the lesion to the nasal and maxillary sinus cavities. Neither has been invaded.

Most of the CBCT machines are structured so that the patient either sits or stands during the exposure, similar to what dental patients have been accustomed to in the past. This differs from virtually all medical CT units in which the patient must assume a supine position. Patients are therefore more comfortable and accepting of the CBCT designs. In addition, because the patient is positioned in a relatively natural head position, the temporomandibular joints can be more accurately evaluated.

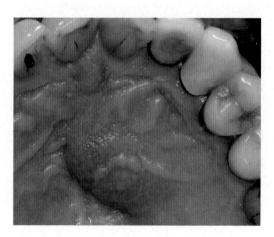

Fig. 4. Case 2. Clinical view of left palatal swelling.

02/19/2007   02/21/2007

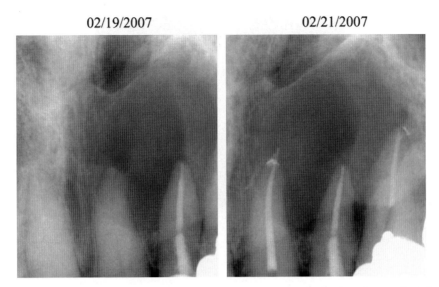

Fig. 5. Case 2. Periapical radiographs of maxillary left incisor teeth showing a large periapical radiolucency. (*Courtesy of* Martin D. Levin, DMD and Chevy Chase, MD.)

Cone beam computed tomography compared with plain film tomography

As compared with plain film tomograms, CBCT technology requires less time for the images to be captured, which is useful for patients who are not comfortable or are unable to keep still. In addition, the images generated via CBCT are less distorted and give the practitioner a better understanding of the density of the bone being imaged.

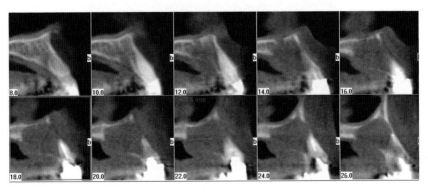

Fig. 6. Case 2. Cross-sectional views showing destruction of the labial and palatal plates and a small area of destruction of the nasal floor.

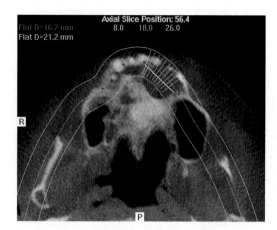

Fig. 7. Case 2. Axial view demonstrating the anteroposterior and lateral extents of osseous destruction measuring 1.6 × 2.1 cm.

Cone beam computed tomography compared with panoramic radiography

While panoramic radiography has been the workhorse for most dental and oral and maxillofacial surgery practices, the images generated do have some shortcomings. Only flat, two dimensional, supero-inferior or postero-anterior images are created. And, as is typical with plain film radiography, panoramic x-rays suffer from superimposition of all structures that lie in the path between the x-ray source and the film or detector. CBCT allows these anatomic entities to be viewed in three dimensions and be included or excluded in the final image by simple digital manipulation. Furthermore, panoramic images are both distorted and magnified, which

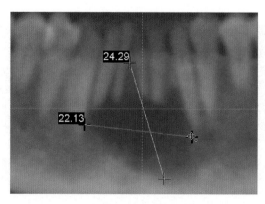

Fig. 8. Case 3. Central giant cell granuloma, mandible. Radiolucent lesion of anterior mandible, 2.2 × 2.4 cm. Patient was asymptomatic.

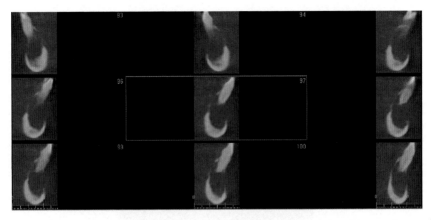

Fig. 9. Case 3. Central giant cell granuloma, mandible. Cross-sectional views illustrate destruction of the labial and lingual plates of bone and blunting of some of the roots.

means that unreliable results are produced when measuring distance on panoramic x-rays, even when the magnification factor is known. Another advantage of CBCT is that it creates images that are both dimensionally faithful as well as anatomically accurate.

CBCT can also be teamed with stereolithographic model construction, which can be used in conjunction with dental implant placement or in the reconstruction of jaws resected due to pathology.

Cone beam computed tomography use in dentistry

CBCT technology allows the dental practitioner to virtually immediately, in her or his office, evaluate patients for a wide variety of maladies, ranging

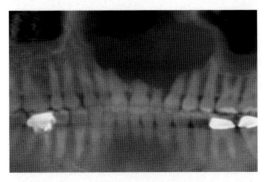

Fig. 10. Case 4. Radiolucent lesion of anterior maxilla, 4.5 × 2.8 cm. Note marked resorption of maxillary left central and lateral incisor (teeth #9 and 10). Patient was asymptomatic.

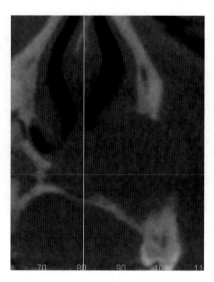

Fig. 11. Case 4. Coronal image, at about the level of a left maxillary premolar shows significant destruction of the body of the maxilla, the lateral wall and the lesion bulging into the nasal cavity.

from dental and jaw trauma and infections, edentulism (quantitative and qualitative osseous evaluation for dental implants), temporomandibular joint osseous pathology, impacted and supernumerary teeth, developmental and congenital jaw deformities, dental endodontic lesions, and oral and maxillofacial pathology.

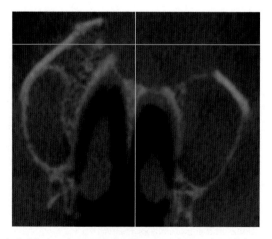

Fig. 12. Case 4. Axial view demonstrating the gross destruction of the anterior maxilla.

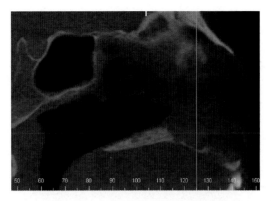

Fig. 13. Case 4. Sagittal midline view reveals the tumor mass and scalloping of the superior aspect of the palatal bone.

It is clear that CBCT is an imaging modality that is becoming an integral part of many dental practices. While much of the early focus has been on its use in dental implantology, it has proven to be a valuable asset in the diagnostic assessment of oral and maxillofacial pathology. The remainder of this article will focus on examples of common as well as some rarely encountered lesions.

Case studies

There is no better way to illustrate the utility of cone beam computed radiography than to demonstrate a variety of oral and maxillofacial pathology cases in which its use assists in the diagnosis and helps to guide the

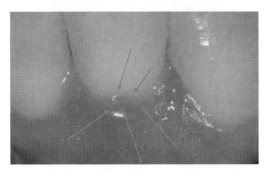

Fig. 14. Case 5. Clinical photograph of noncarious resorption on the labial of the mandibular left lateral incisor tooth. (*Courtesy of* Michael Pascal, DDS, Washington, DC.)

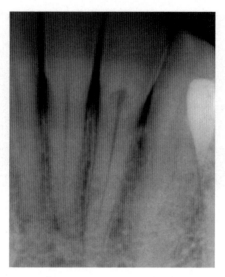

Fig. 15. Case 5. Periapical radiograph illustrating round radiolucency corresponding to labial defect shown in Fig. 14.

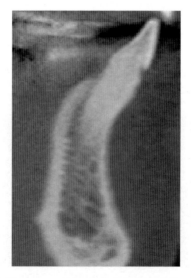

Fig. 16. Case 5. High-definition cross-sectional view of tooth, indicating that the defect extends into the dentin but is well away from the pulp chamber.

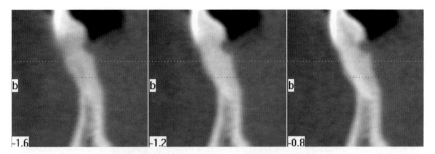

Fig. 17. Case 6. High-definition cross-sectional views of lingual external resorption and caries extending into the pulp chamber.

treatment. Viewing the disease processes in three dimensions provides the practitioner with a more global view of their pathogenesis and extent.

Case 1

Clinical Correlation: The lesion was excised and biopsied Figs. 1–3. Apicoectomy with root end restoration and grafting of the site was accomplished.

Diagnosis: Periapical radicular cyst.

Case 2

Clinical Correlation: The lesion was excised and biopsied Figs. 4–7. Apicoectomy of the maxillary left central incisor followed by grafting the defect with 4 mL of allogeneic bone was performed.

Diagnosis: Periapical radicular cyst.

Case 3

Clinical Correlation: The teeth were nonmobile and the teeth within the lesion all tested vital Figs. 8 and 9. A deep bone biopsy was performed along

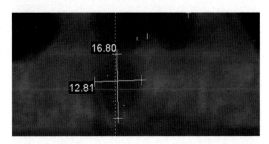

Fig. 18. Case 7. Detail of a panoramic view of the anterior maxilla revealing a well-demarcated radiolucent lesion, 1.3 × 1.7 cm.

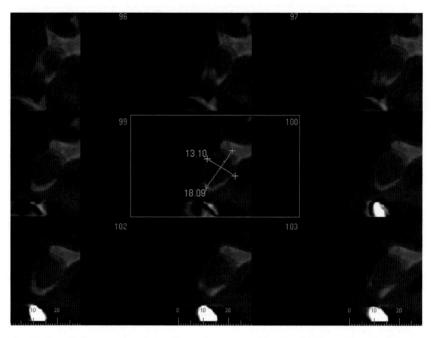

Fig. 19. Case 7. Cross-sectional view illustrating a smooth bordered lesion with mild expansion of the labial and palatal osseous plates.

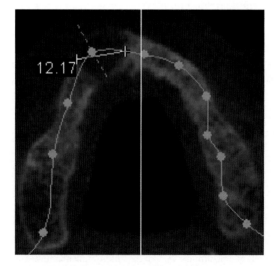

Fig. 20. Case 7. Axial view of same lesion.

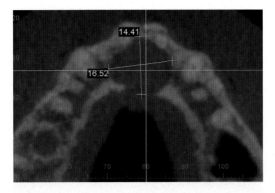

Fig. 21. Case 8. Axial view of radiolucency underlying swollen papilla palatinus.

with an extensive curettage of the lesion. Once the histologic diagnosis was made, the patient was advised of the necessity to perform additional surgery, including removal of some of the teeth, which would prevent adequate excision if left. The patient refused, and on follow-up 10 months later, recurrence was noted.

Diagnosis: Central giant cell granuloma, mandible.

Case 4

Clinical Correlation: Teeth #9 and 10 were nonvital Figs. 10–13. Aspiration of the lesion revealed a solid mass. There was no aspiration of blood or purulence. The patient refused treatment at the time. At a later date, her lesion was biopsied by a colleague who informed me of the diagnosis.

Diagnosis: Central giant cell granuloma, maxilla.

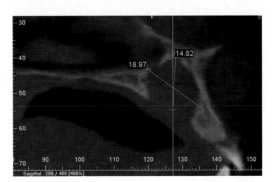

Fig. 22. Case 8. Sagittal view of same lesion illustrating its large dimensions.

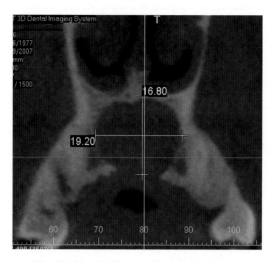

Fig. 23. Case 8. Coronal view of same lesion.

Case 5

Clinical Correlation: This patient was referred specifically for the cross-sectional view to judge the depth of the resorptive defect Figs. 14–16. Because of the information gained, this patient had a restorative procedure performed, but not an endodontic treatment, which had been contemplated.

Diagnosis: External resorption.

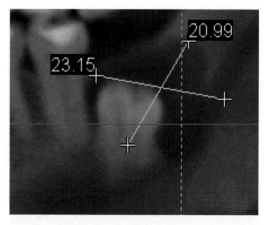

Fig. 24. Case 9. Impacted tooth with dentigerous cyst. Panoramic detail of impacted mandibular left third molar and surrounding radiolucent lesion.

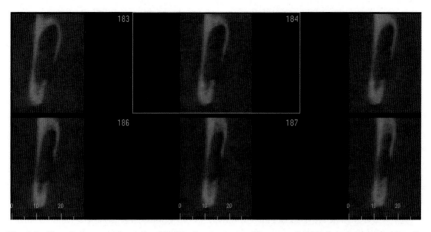

Fig. 25. Case 9. Impacted tooth with dentigerous cyst. Cross-sectional view demonstrating dehiscence of the lingual plate due to the lesion as well as the location of the inferior alveolar nerve canal at the inferior aspect of the mandible.

Case 6

Clinical Correlation: There were no caries associated with the defect Fig. 17. The disease process in this tooth was thought to be too advanced and nonrestorable unless endodontic therapy and forced eruption were undertaken. Based on the cross-sectional CBCT view, the patient decided on extraction and immediate placement of an endosseous implant. This,

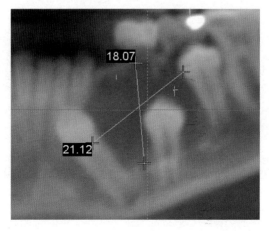

Fig. 26. Case 10. Detail from panoramic view of a 1.8 × 2.1-cm radiolucency of the left mandible. Note the unerupted and impacted teeth and the migration from their normal position in the jaw.

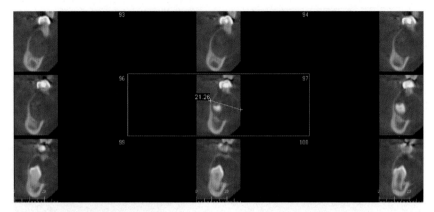

Fig. 27. Case 10. The cross-sectional view illustrates the lesion's smooth borders and significant expansion of the buccal plate giving the lesion an overall width of 2.1 cm. Thinning of the lingual plate can also be appreciated.

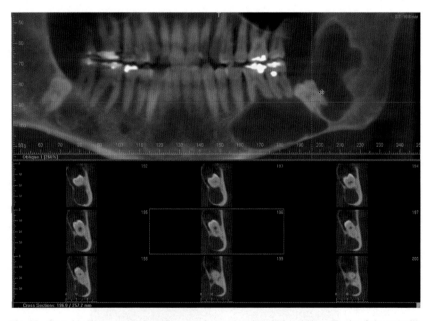

Fig. 28. Case 11. Panoramic view above and cross-sectional view below. Both of the mandibular third molar teeth are impacted. On the left side of the mandible one can appreciate a 7-cm multilocular radiolucency that is focused on in the cross-sectional frames below. Those images reveal a dehiscence of the lingual plate. Note the absence of the inferior alveolar nerve canal on the left. On the right side, one can appreciate another radiolucency, this one 2 cm in diameter predominantly anterior to the impacted molar and inferior to the second molar.

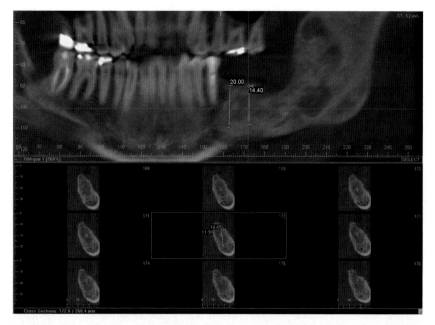

Fig. 29. Case 11. Same views as in Fig. 28 after 13 months of healing. Note the overall healing of the jawbone and in the cross-sectional views, the reformation of the inferior alveolar nerve canal.

as well as placement of a ceramic abutment and an immediate crown, were successfully accomplished.

Diagnosis: External resorption.

Case 7

Clinical Correlation: The cyst was vigorously curetted from the underlying bone and submitted for histopathologic examination Figs. 18–20. The defect was grafted with allogeneic bone. Follow-up examination and radiographs revealed complete resolution without recurrence.

Diagnosis: Residual radicular cyst.

Case 8

Clinical Correlation: The cyst was excised and the defect was grafted with allogeneic bone Figs. 21–23.

Diagnosis: Incisive canal (nasopalatine duct) cyst.

Case 9

Clinical Correlation: The impacted molar was removed, and the cyst was excised and biopsied Figs. 24 and 25. The site was reconstructed with an

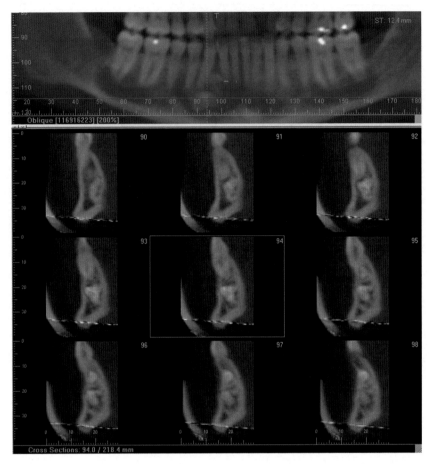

Fig. 30. Case 12. Panoramic view above and cross-sectional view below. The panoramic view shows a lesion composed of radiopaque masses that are somewhat indiscreet. The cross-sectional image reveals that some of the opacities have a form resembling small teeth, while others are just globules of material having a density similar to enamel and dentin. In addition, the lesion is noted to not impinge on the area of the mental foramen or inferior alveolar nerve canal. However, the incisive canal can be seen at the infero-lateral portion of the mandible in the cross-sectional images.

allogeneic bone graft. Knowing the location of the inferior alveolar nerve before surgery helped to avoid injury to it during surgery, resulting in a patient without a postoperative neuropraxia.

Diagnosis: Impacted tooth with dentigerous cyst.

Case 10

Clinical Correlation: The deciduous left mandibular cuspid and first and second molar teeth were removed from this 11-year-old boy Figs. 26 and 27.

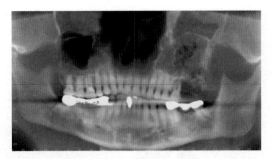

Fig. 31. Case 13. Panoramic view illustrates significant bone loss in the left posterior maxilla, which could interpreted as advanced chronic periodontitis. The maxillary left first molar appears to be floating in a bed of soft tissue.

Cystic tissue was curetted from the crypt and submitted for histopathologic examination. The wound was packed open with iodoform gauze, which was removed slowly over a period of 3 weeks. Within 4 months, the premolar teeth were visible in the mouth, partially erupted. The cuspid had moved superiorly from the inferior border of the mandible but was blocked from complete eruption because of lack of arch space. He was referred for orthodontic therapy.

Diagnosis: Impacted teeth with dentigerous cyst.

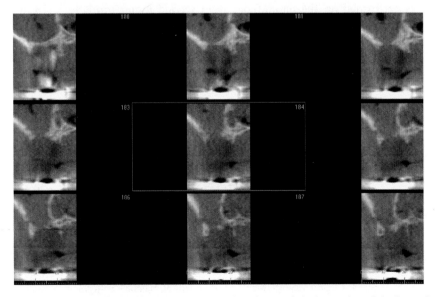

Fig. 32. Case 13. Cross-sectional view demonstrating characteristic destruction of the floor of the maxillary sinus. Relative opacity of the inferior aspect of the sinus can also be appreciated.

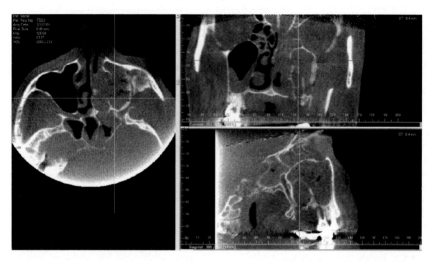

Fig. 33. Case 13. Axial, coronal, and sagittal views demonstrate nearly total opacification of the left maxillary, left ethmoidal, and bilateral frontal sinuses. Destruction of the medial wall of the left maxillary sinus with diseased tissue occupying the left nasal cavity is also noted. In comparison, the right (healthier) maxillary and ethmoidal sinuses are well aerated and appear characteristically radiolucent.

Case 11

Clinical Correlation: Before surgical intervention, endodontic therapy was performed on the mandibular right second molar tooth Figs. 28 and 29. This was done because its devitalization was anticipated during removal of the impacted third molar and the associated cyst. On the left, the decision was made to remove the first and second molars because they would be

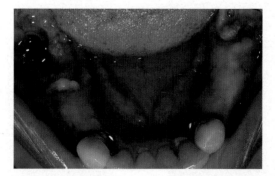

Fig. 34. Case 14. Clinical view showing alveolar ridges of mandible with the destruction of overlying mucosa and exposure of necrotic bone that lies beneath it. These findings are characteristic for this disease process.

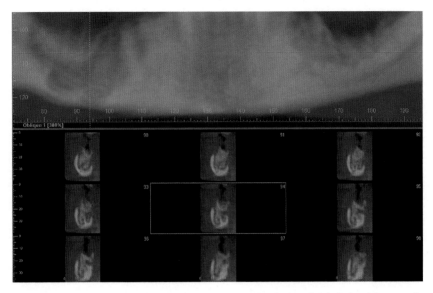

Fig. 35. Case 14. Panoramic view above and cross-sectional view through the right posterior mandible below the mandible seen in Fig. 34. The necrotic bone on each side appears hypodense as compared with the normal living bone of the jaw. The cross-sections exhibit this dead bone to be distinct from the cortical bone of the inferior, buccal, and lingual cortices.

unsupported by any bone following the surgery necessary to appropriately remove the lesion.

In the hospital, the teeth were removed and the cysts were enucleated with care to preserve the inferior alveolar nerves on both sides. Cancellous marrow was harvested from the hip and grafted to each site. The patient is now being restored with endosseous implants.

Diagnosis: Impacted teeth with dentigerous cysts.

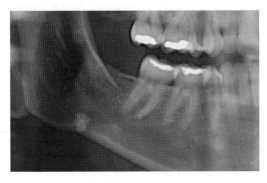

Fig. 36. Case 15. Detail from panoramic view of right mandible revealing a radiopacity located at inferior border in the antegonial region.

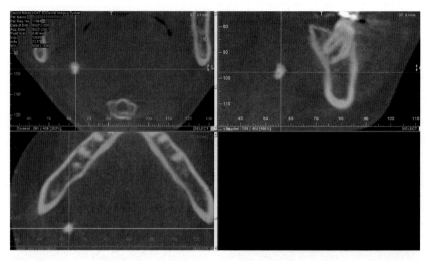

Fig. 37. Case 15. Axial, coronal, and sagittal views establishing that the opacity is located medial to the mandible in the soft tissues of the neck, corresponding to the hilum of the right submaxillary salivary gland.

Case 12

Clinical Correlation: Understanding the nature of the lesion and its relation to important anatomic landmarks (neurovascular bundle and tooth roots) allowed the odontoma to be removed without incident or sequelae Fig. 30. The alveolar volume was restored with an allogeneic graft.

Diagnosis: Compound-complex odontoma.

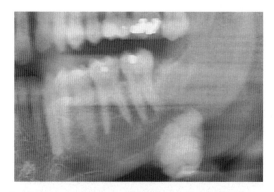

Fig. 38. Case 16. Detail from panoramic view of left mandible revealing a radiopacity located at the inferior border in the antegonial region. Note the similarity in location and density as compared with the lesion presented in the previous case.

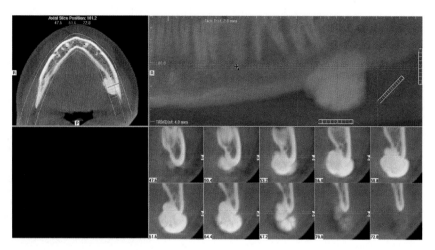

Fig. 39. Case 16. Axial, panoramic, and cross-sectional views indicate that the mass is attached to the inferior and medial aspect of the mandible. The inferior alveolar nerve canal is clearly visible in the cross-sectional views.

Case 13

Clinical Correlation: This patient suffered from multiple myeloma and was treated with intravenous pamidronate disodium, a bisphosphonate drug used commonly to treat this disease Figs. 31–33. He presented with pain and mobility of the maxillary left first molar tooth. The tooth was extracted and surrounding tissue harvested for histopathologic examination confirming the clinical impression of bisphosphonate-related osteonecrosis of the jaws (BRONJ).

Diagnosis: BRONJ involving the maxilla.

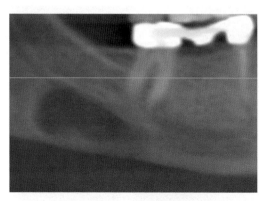

Fig. 40. Case 17. Detail from panoramic view of right posterior mandible demonstrates a large, smooth-bordered radiolucency located inferior to the inferior alveolar nerve canal.

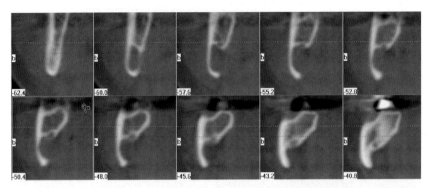

Fig. 41. Case 17. Cross-sectional views through the right mandible reveal a lingual mandibular depression. Note the position of the inferior alveolar nerve canal, just superior to the indentation. This presentation is consistent with a lateral dislocation of the submandibular gland.

Case 14

Clinical Correlation: This woman was also being treated for multiple myeloma, but with a different intravenous bisphosphonate, zoledronic acid Figs. 34 and 35.

Diagnosis: BRONJ of the mandible.

Case 15

Clinical Correlation: The opacity was an incidental finding during a routing dental examination Figs. 36 and 37. The patient, who was totally asymptomatic, had been referred for diagnosis and treatment. The CBCT help to confirm the clinical diagnosis and no treatment was indicated or performed.

Diagnosis: Sialolith, right submaxillary (submandibular) salivary gland.

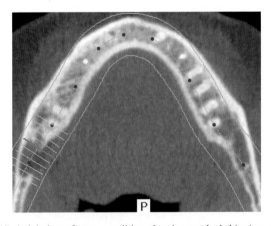

Fig. 42. Case 17. Axial view of same condition showing marked thinning of the mandible.

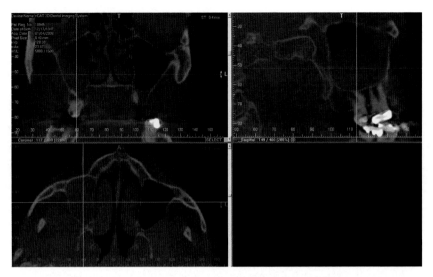

Fig. 43. Case 18. Coronal, axial, and sagittal views of the maxillary sinuses, focusing on the right, illustrating the partial opacification of the right side. Compare with the healthy, completely air-filled, radiolucent left sinus. The ethmoid sinuses are clear bilaterally.

Case 16

Clinical Correlation: This gentleman came to the office for a second opinion Figs. 38 and 39. He was having pain from the slowly enlarging growth beneath his left jaw. He had seen another surgeon who had a fan beam CT performed in a medical facility. It was read by the medical radiologist as a sialolith (stone) of the left submaxillary gland. Since the patient was symptomatic, he was scheduled for surgery to remove his gland. Once the correct diagnosis was achieved through the use of the CBCT, the proper surgery, removal of the osteoma, was accomplished, and the patient became asymptomatic.

Diagnosis: Osteoma, left mandible.

Case 17

Clinical Correlation: This "lesion" does not require treatment Figs. 40–42. A caveat is that any neoplasm that can affect a salivary gland could

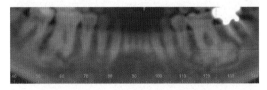

Fig. 44. Case 19. Panoramic view displaying mixed radiolucent-radiopaque well-defined lesions in the areas of the roots of the mandibular right and left first molar teeth.

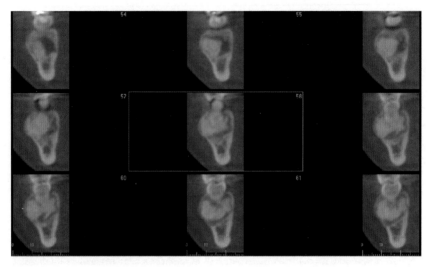

Fig. 45. Case 19. Cross-sectional images through the right mandible, showing the lesion and its expansion of the jaw.

arise in the tissue that occupies the depression and change the appearance of the defect. So, if there is an alteration in its presentation, further investigation is warranted.

Diagnosis: Stafne's bone defect, right mandible.

Case 18

Clinical Correlation: Patients may occasionally present to the dentist, complaining of a toothache, when, in fact, orodental clinical and

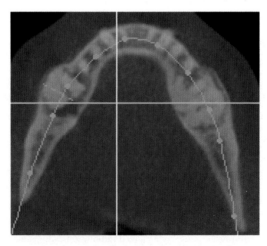

Fig. 46. Case 19. Axial view showing expansion of mandible bilaterally.

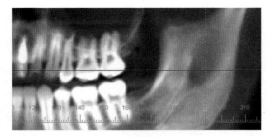

Fig. 47. Case 20. Detail of panoramic view of left mandibular ramus showing what appears to be a tumor of the left mandibular canal at the level of the lingula.

radiographic examinations reveal no odontogenic etiology Fig. 43. In many cases, the problem, as was the case with this individual, is due to disease of the maxillary sinus, which should then be investigated and treated. Our medical colleagues sometimes encounter the reverse situation when patients seek their care for sinus disease, and the problem is actually due to a maxillary tooth.

Diagnosis: Right maxillary sinusitis.

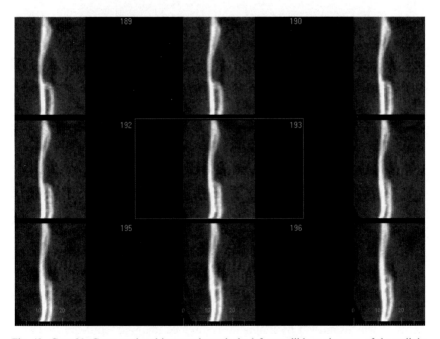

Fig. 48. Case 20. Cross-sectional images through the left mandible at the area of the radiolucency, showing thinning of the jaw. While CBCT is not used primarily for evaluation of soft tissue density, one can note the increased lucency of the soft tissue adjacent to the depression. (Note, because of the software that was used with this particular CBCT at the time the image was taken, the cross-sectional views were always presented in this fashion regardless of the side that was being viewed. The view presented is that of the left mandible.)

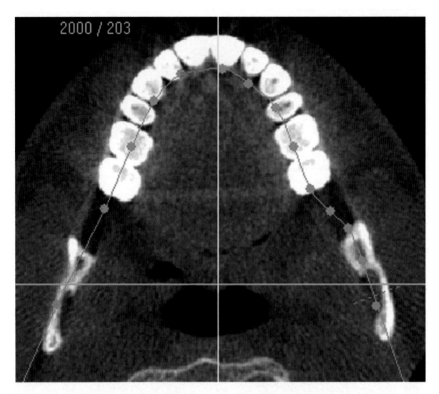

Fig. 49. Case 20. Axial view confirming depression of the left mandibular ramus, medial cortex.

Case 19

Clinical Correlation: This is a fibro-osseous pathologic entity that typically affects the molar regions of middle-aged women, primarily of African heritage, and ordinarily do not require treatment Figs. 44–46. However, there are some patients who, although asymptomatic, wish to have a definitive histologic diagnosis. Deep bone biopsy was performed on one of the lesions confirming its identity.

Diagnosis: Florid cemento-osseous dysplasia.

Case 20

Clinical Correlation: Because of the unusual radiographic appearance, the mass was examined by magnetic resonance imaging, confirming that it was abnormal tissue Figs. 47–49. Therefore, the lesion was excised via an intraoral approach along the ascending ramus. Histologic examination confirmed the clinical diagnosis of lipoma.

Diagnosis: Lipoma mimicking neoplasm within the mandibular canal.

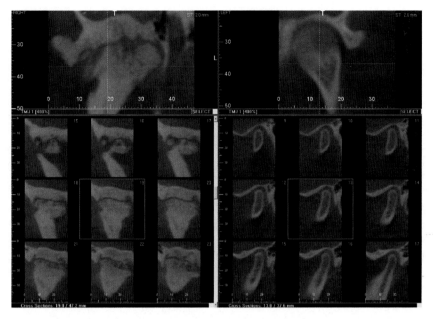

Fig. 50. Case 21. Sagittal and coronal images demonstrate vast abnormality of the right condylar head and glenoid fossa. There is flattening of the condyle with pitting of the surface and osteophyte formation. The roof of the glenoid fossa is markedly thickened. Compare the right joint to the osseous structure of the normal left temporomandibular joint.

Case 21

Clinical Correlation: This is the joint of a otherwise healthy 33-year-old male who has no history of trauma or other diseases that could affect the temporomandibular joint Fig. 50. He sought treatment because of worsening pain not controlled by medications and limitation of jaw motion. The problem had begun a few years previously and had become considerably worse in during the 5 months before presentation at the office. Technetium-99 (Tc-99) bone scanning showed increased uptake at the joint indicating that the destructive process was still ongoing.

Treatment consisted of condylectomy, osteoplasty of the glenoid fossa, and immediate joint reconstruction with a costochondral rib graft.

Diagnosis: Severe osteoarthritis of right temporomandibular joint.

Case 22

Clinical Correlation: Fifteen years before presentation, the patient had histologically diagnosed fibrous dysplasia of the left maxilla and mandible, which was surgically reduced for cosmesis Figs. 51 and 52. He presented to

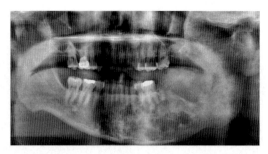

Fig. 51. Case 22. Panoramic radiograph displays gross enlargement of the mandible with soap bubble radiolucencies extending from the right parasymphysis to the left mandibular body.

our office because he had noticed a sudden increase in his left facial swelling. Following incisional biopsy and establishment of the diagnosis, the neo- plasm was treated initially with chemotherapy to shrink the tumor mass. This was followed by surgical excision, then reconstruction with a composite vascularized graft.

Diagnosis: Spindle cell sarcoma of left mandible.

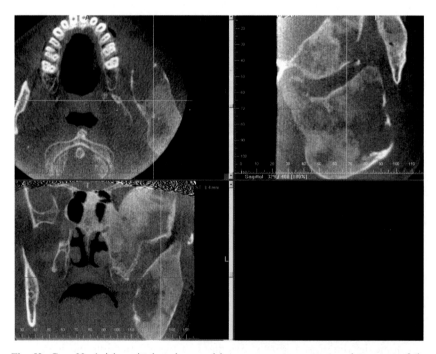

Fig. 52. Case 22. Axial, sagittal, and coronal images present a more complete extent of the lesion, showing its penetration to include the complete ramus, coronoid process, and condyle, as well as the maxilla and malar bone.

Summary

It is clear that the dental profession has entered a new age of radiographic diagnostic imaging. As has been shown through a number of examples, being able to visualize oral and maxillofacial pathologic entities in three dimensions assists in the diagnosis as well as in planning the appropriate treatment. The technology is an improvement for our profession and for the patients it serves.

ELSEVIER
SAUNDERS

THE DENTAL
CLINICS
OF NORTH AMERICA

Dent Clin N Am 52 (2008) 875–890

Contemporary Imaging of the Temporomandibular Joint

Emma L. Lewis, BDS, MBBS*,
M. Franklin Dolwick, DMD, PhD,
Shelly Abramowicz, DMD,
Stephanie L. Reeder, DMD

*Department of Oral and Maxillofacial Surgery, University of Florida College of Dentistry,
Health Science Center, P.O. Box 100416, Gainesville, FL 32610-0416, USA*

Imaging modalities of the temporomandibular joint (TMJ) have continued to evolve during the past decade. With the advent of newer techniques and computer enhancements, TMJ imaging has enabled a better appreciation for TMJ anatomy and function. Correlation of these images with clinical findings has led to an improved understanding of the pathophysiology of TMJ disorders. As our understanding of TMJ disorders progresses, the development of new treatment algorithms will ensue. Current management of TMJ disorders relies heavily on clinical evaluation, with minor influence from information obtained through TMJ imaging. Although TMJ imaging in a clinical setting may have declined, it still has an expanding role at the research level in the quest for greater understanding of this complex group of joint disorders [1].

The goals for TMJ imaging include evaluating the integrity of the structures when disease is suspected, determining the extent of disease or monitoring its progression when disease is present, and evaluating the effects of treatment. Specific anatomic areas of the TMJ include the mandibular condyle, the glenoid fossa, the articular eminences of the temporal bone, and the soft tissue components of the articular disk, its attachments, and the joint cavity.

---

* Corresponding author. Department of Oral and Maxillofacial Surgery, University of Florida College of Dentistry, Health Science Center, P.O. Box 100416, Gainesville, FL 32610-0416.

E-mail address: elewis@dental.ufl.edu (E.L. Lewis).

0011-8532/08/$ - see front matter © 2008 Elsevier Inc. All rights reserved.
doi:10.1016/j.cden.2008.06.001
dental.theclinics.com

As with any laboratory test or imaging, clear indications should be established to justify the test. The need for TMJ imaging should be determined at an individual level after taking a thorough history and performing an appropriate clinical examination of the patient. The symptoms and signs presented should guide a practitioner to develop a differential diagnosis of possible TMJ pathology. Based on the differential diagnosis, the most appropriate mode of imaging should then be ordered, with consideration given to how the image results will influence overall management. Other factors that should be considered when determining the appropriate mode of imaging include the likelihood of hard or soft tissue pathology, the availability of specialized equipment, the cost of the examination, the amount of radiation exposure, and any contraindications, such as allergy to intravenous contrast agents or pregnancy. The efficacy of the technique will be determined by the quality of the image obtained combined with the skills of the person interpreting the image.

This article reviews the various techniques available for imaging the TMJ, with emphasis on contemporary imaging modalities, and includes a discussion of the method, indications, advantages, and limitations. The following techniques are included: plain film radiography, tomography, panoramic radiology, arthrography, ultrasonography, CT, MRI, and nuclear imaging.

Plain film radiography

Plain films refer to X rays made with a stationary x-ray source and film. Plain films of the TMJ depict only mineralized parts of the joint, such as bone; they do not give any information about nonmineralized cartilage, soft tissues, or the presence of joint effusion. Radiographic changes are often not seen until a sufficient volume of destruction or alteration in bone mineral content has occurred [2]. Plain films are also limited by the superimposition of adjacent structures, which can make visualizing all parts of the joint difficult. To overcome this limitation, multiple plain film techniques have been developed to image the joint from various angles. Plain films are the least expensive and require simple equipment that is often available in the dental office. Although many of these techniques have been superseded by CT, which offers superior anatomic visualization of joint structures, several plain film views have traditionally been used to image the TMJ and have contributed to our diagnosis and treatment of TMJ disorders.

Transcranial view

The introduction of the transcranial view of the TMJ is attributed to Schuller in 1905. In this lateral oblique transcranial projection, the x-ray beam is directed parallel to the long axis of the condyle. At this angulation, the cranial bones are the only structures superimposed over the joint. As a result, a sharp image of the mandibular condyle, articular eminence, and glenoid fossa is obtained (Fig. 1). The transcranial view shows mainly the lateral part of the joint and can be used to determine condylar position and size, depth of the fossa, slope of the eminence, and width of the joint space.

Transmaxillary view

In the transmaxillary view technique, the x-ray beam is directed perpendicular to the long axis of the condyle. Changing the vertical and horizontal orientation helps with condyle and mastoid process superimposition. The lower jaw is also protruded to avoid superimposition of the condyle onto the base of the skull. This view, along with the transcranial view, provides a three-dimensional evaluation of the condyle for fractures, severe degenerative joint disease, and neoplasms.

Submentovertex view

The submentovertex view directs the x-ray beam through the chin region parallel to the posterior border of the ramus toward the base of the skull. This view shows the angulations of the long axes of the condyles relative to a line drawn between the auditory canals and the cephalostat ear rods (if used to position the patient), or to a perpendicular midsagittal line. This view is a useful supplement to examine condylar displacement and rotation in the horizontal plane associated with trauma or facial asymmetry. Because the patient is positioned with full neck extension, this technique is contraindicated in trauma patients who are suspected of neck injury.

Other views

The transpharyngeal view involves placing the x-ray tube close to the contralateral joint and aiming the beam toward the opposite joint, which is adjacent to the film. As a result, the joint nearer the film is in focus, whereas the joint closest to the x-ray source appears out of focus. This

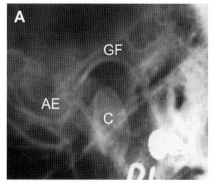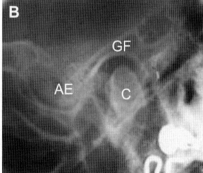

Fig. 1. (*A, B*) Lateral transcranial view of TMJ in open mouth and closed mouth positions. AE, articular eminence; C, condyle; GF, glenoid fossa.

projection provides an acceptable view of the TMJ, condylar neck, mandibular ramus, and zygomatic region.

The Reverse Towne's projection positions the patient's forehead directly against the film. The patient is then instructed to open his/her mouth to bring the condylar head out of the glenoid fossa, thus reducing the superimposition of these structures on one another. The x-ray beam is then positioned behind the patient's occiput at a 30° angle to the horizontal and centered on the condyles. This projection offers an excellent view of the condylar neck and is useful in the trauma setting when a condylar fracture is suspected [3–5].

Posterior-anterior and lateral cephalograms give little information about the TMJ itself because of the superimposition of adjacent bony structures. However, they can be used for serial examinations of patients who have skeletal asymmetry.

With the increasing use and availability of CT and cone-beam CT, the use of plain films for imaging the hard tissues of the TMJ is becoming less popular.

Conventional tomography

Tomography is a radiographic technique that clearly depicts a specific slice or section of the patient. Understanding the concept of sectional images is important because it has become the basis for many modern imaging techniques we use today, such as panoramic radiography and CT. In conventional tomography, the x-ray source and film simultaneously move around a fixed rotation point in opposite directions. Objects lying within a specific plane of interest are seen in focus, whereas those structures outside the predetermined focal plane appear blurred. Varying patterns of tomographic movement, or rotation, can be performed to ensure the clearest view of the bony components of the TMJ and to reduce the problem of superimposition. The disadvantages of tomography include the inability to evaluate soft tissue and the fact that the required equipment is more expensive than a conventional x-ray machine. With the advent of CT and MRI, which have superior low-contrast resolution, conventional film tomography is used less frequently.

Panoramic radiography

This imaging technique is one of the most commonly used by dentists and dental specialists. The fundamental principle behind panoramic radiography is based on the tomographic concept of imaging a section of the body while blurring images outside the desired plane. The x-ray source and film are set opposite to each other and rotate around the whole head with a narrow focal trough so that the TMJs and teeth are in focus, but the adjacent structures are blurred. The narrow focal trough is produced by lead collimators in the shape of a slit located at the x-ray source and the film. The size and shape of the focal trough and the number of rotation centers vary with the manufacturer of the panoramic unit.

Panoramic radiography is a useful screening technique for condylar abnormalities such as erosions, sclerosis, osteophyte formation, resorption, and fractures (Fig. 2). In addition, the panoramic film also gives information about the teeth, mandible, and maxilla, which may help with the overall diagnosis by ruling out odontogenic sources or other pathology of the jaws. However, a disadvantage of panoramic radiography is that the glenoid fossa and articular eminences are not well visualized because of the superimposition of the base of the skull and zygomatic arches. Condylar position also cannot be evaluated because the mouth is slightly open and protruded during this view [3–5].

Arthrography

Arthrography is an imaging method by which radiopaque contrast dye is injected into the lower TMJ spaces under fluoroscopic guidance to image the soft tissue structures. Katzberg and colleagues [6] introduced this modified arthrotomographic technique for TMJ imaging in 1979. Before this, plain films and conventional tomography were the only methods available for imaging the TMJ. In contrast to the previous imaging techniques, which were static views of the joint, arthrography was the first dynamic study of the joint [7]. According to the pattern by which the contrast agent flows, adhesions, disk perforations, and disk function can be studied during open and closing movements. This technique is ideal for small disk perforations and for visualizing the movement of the joints.

The disadvantages of arthrography are that it is an invasive procedure, requiring insertion of a needle into the TMJ by a skilled operator, which may result in complications, such as bleeding and introduction of infection. Another disadvantage is the potential for an allergic reaction to the contrast agent and the high radiation exposure. The fact that a needle is inserted into the joint under anesthesia does, however, afford the operator the opportunity to perform a simultaneous arthrocentesis so that the procedure can be

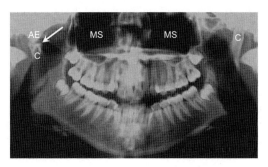

Fig. 2. Panorex. White arrow indicates degenerative changes of right condyle. AE, articular eminence; C, condyle; MS, maxillary sinus.

diagnostic and therapeutic. Arthrography is rarely used today because of its invasiveness and the associated radiation exposure to the patient. Other imaging modalities such as MRI now offer excellent soft tissue depiction without the need for injection of contrast or radiation exposure [5,7].

Ultrasonography

Ultrasonography uses sound waves of high frequency to produce images of the body. As the sound waves travel through the body, they encounter a boundary between tissues of varying densities. Depending on the density, or resistance, of the tissue, reflective echoes are returned to the ultrasound probe at different speeds and relayed to a machine that translates the echoes into a picture.

Ultrasonography has been described in imaging the TMJ with some beneficial, albeit limited, results [8,9]. Most favorable results have been noted in relation to evaluating disk position, with minimal benefit in evaluating hard tissue changes [10–17]. Gateno and colleagues used ultrasonography for intraoperative assessment of condylar position in relation to the glenoid fossa during mandibular ramus osteotomy procedures. Condylar position was identified correctly in 38 of 40 ultrasound images with a sensitivity of 95% [18]. However, later studies using ultrasonography to evaluate condylar erosion and osteoarthritic changes of the condyle found it to be inferior to CT imaging, mainly because of interference by reflective echoes from the glenoid fossa [19–21].

When evaluating TMJ disk position for internal derangement, ultrasonography has shown some benefit, especially when high-resolution, dynamic, real-time ultrasonography is used [12]. However, ultrasonographic evaluation of the TMJ disk position is currently associated with a high number of false-positives, which could ultimately result in overtreatment. Currently, MRI is more accurate and continues to be the gold standard for imaging soft tissue of the TMJ [22].

As advancements in ultrasound probe technology continue, more detailed imaging and improvement in tissue differentiation may contribute to a reduction in the number of false-positives and, therefore, overtreatment. Further research in this imaging modality for the TMJ is needed because ultrasonography offers many advantages, including reduced cost, accessibility, fast results, decreased examination time, and lack of radiation exposure.

CT/cone-beam CT

CT is an imaging method that combines multiple X rays taken at different angles to create cross-sectional images of the body. Each image is considered a "slice" and can be reformatted to create a three-dimensional image of the body [4]. CT has been central to the advancement of diagnostic imaging in the field of medicine. With the recent advent of cone-beam CT, the use of CT imaging in the field of dentistry is becoming integral to the practice of orthodontics, implant dentistry, and oral surgery [23–30]. Cone-beam CT uses a cone-shaped x-ray beam in contrast to the fan-shaped x-ray beam of spiral CT. The beam performs a single rotation around the head of the patient at a constant angle, producing a volumetric data set that is later reconstructed into three-dimensional images. The amount of radiation exposure is smaller and the examination time is shorter, when compared with conventional CT. The current state-of-the-art CT technique is multidetector row CT, in which 16 to 64 detector rows are used along with thin slice profiles, such that volumetric acquisition of data is achieved. Data can then be presented at equal resolution in any plane including the panoramic plane. Reconstruction algorithms and optimal windowing allow for imaging of hard and soft tissue pathology [31].

The application of conventional CT in imaging the TMJ has been most significant in the evaluation of hard tissue or bony changes of the joint. Pathologic changes, such as osteophytes, condylar erosion, fractures, ankylosis, dislocation, and growth abnormalities such as condylar hyperplasia, are optimally viewed on CT (Figs. 3 and 4). Westesson [32] and DeBont [33] found CT to be superior to plain films and MRI for imaging the bony structures of the TMJ. In contrast, Westesson [32] found CT to be less accurate than MRI for imaging the disk. Multidetector row CT can be used to show disk displacement and synovitis, effusions, and erosions [31].

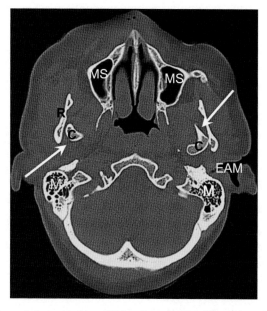

Fig. 3. Axial CT scan in bone windows. White arrows indicate bilateral condyle fractures with anteromedial dislocation. C, condyle; EAM, external auditory meatus; M, mastoid air cells; MS, maxillary sinus; R, ramus.

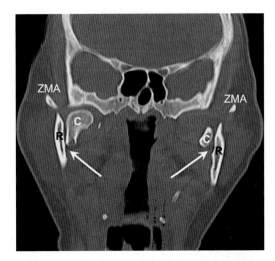

Fig. 4. Coronal CT scan in bone windows. White arrows indicate bilateral condyle fractures with medial displacement. C, condyle; R, ramus; ZMA, zygomatic arch.

The main disadvantages of the use of CT in imaging the TMJ have been radiation exposure, expense, accessibility, and size of the equipment. Cone-beam CT has improved on several of these issues. Less radiation exposure, in-office use, decreased cost, and a more detailed view of the TMJ in the sagittal plane by cone-beam CT has taken this imaging modality in a new direction.

MRI

MRI was first developed in July 1977. MRI uses a powerful magnet, radiowaves, and computer analysis to produce excellent soft tissue images. The magnetic field aligns the magnetization of hydrogen ions within the body, such as those found in fat and water. Radiowaves are used to alter this alignment, which causes the hydrogen ions to emit a weak radio signal that is amplified by the scanner. Additional magnetic fields can then be used to manipulate the signal, to build up information to reconstruct the area of interest. MRI is the most accurate radiographic imaging modality for visualizing TMJ disk position [34] and associated soft tissue structures. The images are presented in T1- and T2-weighted sequences. T1-weighted images are used for visualization of osseous and disk tissues (Fig. 5), whereas T2-weighted images demonstrate inflammation and effusions (Fig. 6). MRI is used to analyze the position of the articular disk in sagittal and coronal planes (Figs. 7 and 8), dynamic assessment of condylar translation and disk movement during opening and closing, disk morphology, joint effusions (Fig. 9), synovitis, osseous erosions, and degenerative joint disease [35,36]. MRI has been widely accepted as a tool for diagnosing

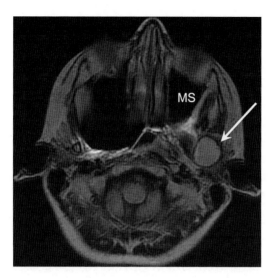

Fig. 5. T1-weighted axial MRI. White arrow indicates cystic lesion of the left condyle with fluid levels. MS, maxillary sinus.

internal derangement and has been reported to be 95% accurate in assessing disk position and form and 93% accurate in assessing osseous changes [37]. MRI helps visualize aspects of TMJ pathology that may help in diagnosing TMJ dysfunction, including thickening of tendon attachments, rupture of retrodiscal tissues, joint effusion, or osteoarthritic changes such as condylar flattening or osteophyte formation. However, the question of whether TMJ

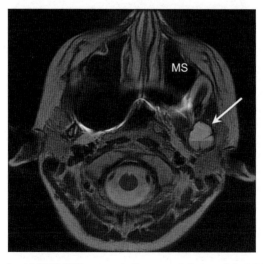

Fig. 6. T2-weighted axial MRI. White arrow indicates cystic lesion of the left condyle with fluid levels. MS, maxillary sinus.

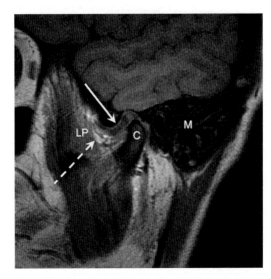

Fig. 7. T1-weighted sagittal MRI of TMJ. Solid white arrow indicates articular disk anteriorly displaced. Broken white arrow indicates a joint effusion. C, condyle; LP, lateral pterygoid; M, mastoid air cells.

disk displacement may be linked to the onset, progression, or cessation of TMJ signs and symptoms remains controversial [38]. Therefore, studies are needed to improve our understanding of the relevance of these radiographic findings as sources of TMJ pain and dysfunction.

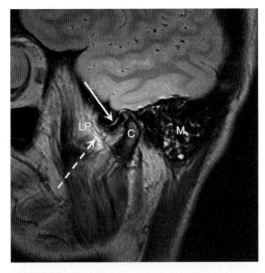

Fig. 8. T2-weighted sagittal view of TMJ. Solid white arrow indicates articular disk anteriorly displaced. Broken white arrow indicates a joint effusion. C, condyle; LP, lateral pterygoid; M, mastoid air cells.

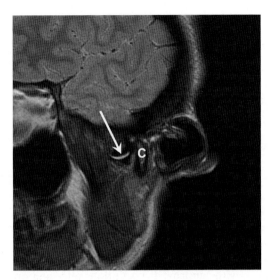

Fig. 9. T2-weighted sagittal MRI. White arrow indicates a joint effusion. C, condyle.

MRI is advantageous because no ionizing radiation is used. However, it requires expensive equipment operated and interpreted by skilled technicians and radiologists. It is also contraindicated in pregnant women and in patients who have implanted metal devices such as pacemakers or aneurysm clips. Titanium dental implants are not a contraindication.

Nuclear medicine

In contrast to the aforementioned imaging modalities, which focus on anatomic integrity, nuclear medicine is unique in that it can assess changes in physiologic function as a direct result of biochemical alterations at the cellular and subcellular level. It is, therefore, used as a physiologic adjunct to the anatomic detail provided by other imaging modalities.

Nuclear medicine uses radionuclide-labeled tracers injected intravenously, which emit gamma radiation. Using a scintillation crystal that fluoresces on interaction with gamma rays, a gamma scintillation camera detects the emitted radiation. The fluorescence is then amplified by a photomultiplier to produce an image. These images are known as radionuclide imaging or nuclear scintigraphy. In bone scintigraphy, such as that used in imaging of the TMJ, the most commonly used radiotracer is technetium diphosphonate, because of its low radiation dose and short half-life. The radiation dose from intravenous injection compares with that of other standard radiographic procedures. Uptake of the radionuclide corresponds with the metabolic activity in the area of the body being examined and depends on local blood flow, vascular permeability, enzymatic action, and the amount of mineralized bone crystals and immature collagen that bind to phosphate.

Since the introduction of nuclear imaging in the early 1950s, technologic advances in the concept of tomography have enabled single-photon emission computed tomography (SPECT) and positron emission tomography (PET) to overcome the disadvantages of image distortion and superimposition associated with planar nuclear imaging. Because the formed image seen in planar nuclear imaging represents radiation emission from a general area rather than a specific anatomic location, nuclear activity from adjacent structures may be superimposed on the area of interest and may present a distorted view.

This disadvantage is similar to the limitation of plain films when compared with CT. Just as CT improved on the one-dimensional view of plain films by using multiple detectors or a single moving detector to acquire multiple transaxial slices, SPECT acquires multiple images or "slices" by rotating the gamma scintillation camera 360° around the patient. These slices can then be stacked to give a three-dimensional representation (axial, coronal, and sagittal) of the distribution of the radionuclide in the patient, providing images with improved resolution and anatomic localization (Figs. 10 and 11). SPECT can also be combined with anatomic data acquired by CT to form functional anatomic mapping. This combination enables early detection and precise location of the bony remodeling and may be a more accurate interpretation than SPECT alone. This combination uses low radiation dose and is highly sensitive and specific when compared with conventional radiography and tomography [4].

A more recent development in nuclear imaging is PET, which is reported to have sensitivity 100 times that of a gamma camera. PET uses positron-emitting

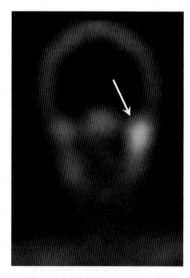

Fig. 10. Coronal view of SPECT bone scan. White arrow indicates increased uptake in the lesion in the left condyle.

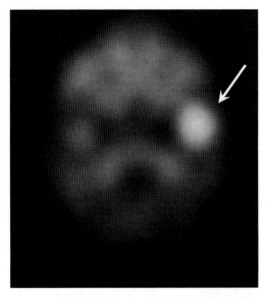

Fig. 11. Axial view of **SPECT** bone scan. White arrow indicates increased uptake in the lesion in the left condyle.

isotopes. When emitted from the tissue, the positrons interact with adjacent electrons to produce two gamma rays traveling in opposite directions. Multiple detectors are placed within the PET scanners and, by a process called annihilation coincidence detection, several gamma emissions can be detected at nearly the same time.

Nuclear imaging in the evaluation of the TMJ is useful when assessing skeletal growth, condylar hyperplasia, synovitis, and the quantification of arthritis in patients who have rheumatoid arthritis or osteoarthritis. Although bone scintigraphy has a high sensitivity for bone metabolism, it also has a low specificity in that it cannot differentiate among conditions such as bone healing, growth, infection, arthritic changes, or tumors. A 10% increase in osteolytic or osteogenic activity can be seen using nuclear imaging compared with the 40% to 50% decalcification needed to occur before changes are identified using conventional radiography [39]. However, the cause of the osteolytic or osteogenic activity cannot be determined from nuclear imaging alone. In addition, nuclear imaging is helpful in determining joint stability before dental rehabilitation, orthodontic therapy, or orthognathic surgery; in diagnosing fibro-osseous lesions, vascular lesions, osteomyelitis, metastatic disease; and in follow-up evaluations of primary tumors [39]. It can also be used in the evaluation of osseous allografts by demonstrating the establishment of blood flow to the grafted area and observing uptake patterns between the remaining jaw and graft site.

The main disadvantages of nuclear imaging of the TMJ include its inability to reveal the morphology of the osseous components or disk displacement and the need for intravenous injection of radioactive pharmaceutics, which results in whole body radiation exposure. Results of nuclear imaging are also nonspecific; however, when used in combination with other imaging modalities, it can be a useful adjunct to aid in diagnosis of metabolic TMJ conditions.

Summary

After a thorough review of the literature, it is clear that multiple imaging modalities are available for evaluation of the TMJ. The need for TMJ imaging should be assessed on an individual basis, depending on the signs and symptoms obtained and the working diagnoses.

Based on the evidence currently available, MRI continues to be the gold standard for imaging disk position and the soft tissues of the TMJ, including joint effusions. In contrast, CT is the ideal imaging choice for evaluating hard tissues, adding improvement in accessibility and radiation dosage with the use of the new cone-beam CT. For more specific TMJ pathology, nuclear imaging is useful in determining if the process is in an active or quiescent phase.

As advancements in this area continue, our understanding of this complex joint and its pathology will follow, which will lead to more defined imaging indications and ultimately, to improved treatment outcomes.

References

[1] Katzberg R. Perspectives on the influence of "arthrotomography of the temporomandibular joint." Am J Roentgenol 2007;188:1553–4.
[2] Epstein JB, Rea A, Chahal O. The use of bone scintigraphy in temporomandibular joint disorders. Oral Dis 2002;8:47–53.
[3] Brooks SL, Brand JW, Gibbs SJ, et al. Imaging of the temporomandibular joint. A position paper of the American Academy of Oral and Maxillofacial Radiology. Oral Surg Oral Med Oral Pathol Oral Radiol Endod 1997;83:609–18.
[4] Frederiksen N. Specialized radiographic techniques. In: White S, Pharoah M, editors. Oral radiology: principles and interpretation. 4th edition. St. Louis (MO): Mosby; 2000. p. 217–40.
[5] Pharoah M, Petrikowski G. Imaging temporomandibular joint disorders. Oral Maxillofac Surg Clin North Am 2001;13:623–38.
[6] Katzberg RW, Dolwick MF, Bales DJ, et al. Arthrotomography of the temporomandibular joint: new technique and preliminary observations. AJR Am J Roentgenol 1979;132:949–55.
[7] Helms CA, Kaplan P. Diagnostic imaging of the temporomandibular joint: recommendations for use of various techniques. Am J Roentgenol 1990;154:319–22.
[8] Nabeih YB, Speculand B. Ultrasonography as a diagnostic aid in temporomandibular dysfunction. A preliminary investigation. Int J Oral Maxillofac Surg 1991;20:182–6.
[9] Stefanoff V, Hausamen JE, van den Berghe P. Ultrasound imaging of the TMJ disc in asymptomatic volunteers. Preliminary report. J Craniomaxillofac Surg 1992;20:337–40.

[10] Emshoff R, Bertram S, Rudisch A, et al. The diagnostic value of ultrasonography to determine the temporomandibular joint disk position. Oral Surg Oral Med Oral Pathol Oral Radiol Endod 1997;84:688–96.

[11] Landes C, Walendzik H, Klein C. Sonography of the temporomandibular joint from 60 examinations and comparison with MRI and axiography. J Craniomaxillofac Surg 2000; 28:352–61.

[12] Jank S, Rudisch A, Bodner G, et al. High-resolution ultrasonography of the TMJ: helpful diagnostic approach for patients with TMJ disorders? J Craniomaxillofac Surg 2001;29: 366–71.

[13] Emshoff R, Jank S, Rudisch A, et al. Are high resolution ulstrasonographic signs of disk displacement valid? J Oral Maxillofac Surg 2002;60:623–8.

[14] Emshoff R, Jank S, Bertram S, et al. Disk displacement of the temporomandibular joint: sonography versus MR imaging. Am J Roentgenol 2002;178:1557–62.

[15] Emshoff R, Jank S, Rudisch A, et al. Error patterns and observer variations in the high-resolution ultrasonography imaging evaluation of the disk position of the temporomandibular joint. Oral Surg Oral Med Oral Pathol Oral Radiol Endod 2002;93:369–75.

[16] Uysal S, Kansu H, Akhan O, et al. Comparison of ultrasonography with magnetic resonance imaging in the diagnosis of temporomandibular joint internal derangments: a preliminary investigation. Oral Surg Oral Med Oral Pathol Oral Radiol Endod 2002;94:115–21.

[17] Landes C, Goral W, Sader R, et al. Three-dimensional versus two-dimensional sonography of the temporomandibular joint in comparison to MRI. Eur J Radiol 2007;61:235–44.

[18] Gateno J, Miloro M, Hendler BH, et al. The use of ultrasound to determine the position of the mandibular condyle. J Oral Maxillofac Surg 1993;51:1081–6.

[19] Emshoff R, Brandlmaier I, Bodner G, et al. Condylar erosion and disc displacement: detection with high-resolution ultrasonography. J Oral Maxillofac Surg 2003;61:877–81.

[20] Tognini F, Manfredini D, Melchioree D, et al. Comparison of ultrasonography and magnetic resonance imaging in the evaluation of temporomandibular joint disc displacement. J Oral Rehabil 2005;32:248–53.

[21] Landes C, Goral W, Mack M, et al. 3-D sonography for diagnosis of osteoarthrosis and disk degeneration of the temporomandibular joint, compared with MRI. Ultrasound Med Biol 2006;32:627–32.

[22] Jank S, Emshoff R, Norer B, et al. Diagnostic quality of dynamic high-resolution ultrasonography of the TMJ—a pilot study. Int J Oral Maxillofac Surg 2005;34:132–7.

[23] Honda K, Larheim TA, Johannessen S, et al. Ortho cubic super-high resolution computed tomography: a new radiographic technique with application to the temporomandibular joint. Oral Surg Oral Med Oral Pathol Oral Radiol Endod 2001;91:239–43.

[24] Hashimoto K, Arai Y, Iwai K, et al. A comparison of a new limited cone beam computed tomography machine for dental use with a multidetector row helical CT machine. Oral Surg Oral Med Oral Pathol Oral Radiol Endod 2003;95:371–7.

[25] Tsiklakis K, Syriopoulos K, Stamatakis HC. Radiographic examination of the temporomandibular joint using cone beam computed tomography. Dentomaxillofac Radiol 2004; 33:196–201.

[26] Honda K, Arai Y, Kashima M, et al. Evaluation of the usefulness of the limited cone beam CT (3DX) in the assessment of the thickness of the roof of the glenoid fossa of the temporomandibular joint. Dentomaxillofac Radiol 2004;33:391–5.

[27] Hilgers M, Scarfe W, Scheetz J, et al. Accuracy of linear temporomandibular joint measurements with cone beam computed tomography and digital cephalometric radiography. Am J Orthod Dentofacial Orthop 2005;128:803–11.

[28] Honda L, Larheim TA, Maruhashi K, et al. Osseous abnormalities of the mandibular condyle: diagnostic reliability of cone beam computed tomography compared with helical computed tomography based on autopsy material. Dentomaxillofac Radiol 2006;35:152–7.

[29] Hintze H, Wiese M, Wenzel A. Cone beam CT and conventional tomography for the detection of morphological temporomandibular joint changes. Dentomaxillofac Radiol 2007;36:192–7.

[30] Honey O, Scarfe W, Hilgers M, et al. Accuracy of cone beam computed tomography imaging of the temporomandibular joint: comparisons with panoramic radiology and linear tomography. Am J Orthod Dentofacial Orthop 2007;132:429–38.

[31] Boeddinghaus R, Whyte A. Current concepts in maxillofacial imaging. Eur J Radiol 2008; 66(3):396–418.

[32] Westesson P, Katzburg R, Sanchez-Woodworth R, et al. CT and MR of the temporomandibular joint: comparison with autopsy specimens. Am J Roentgenol 1987;148:1165–71.

[33] DeBont L, Van der Kuijl B, Stegenga L, et al. Computed tomography in differential diagnosis of temporomandibular joint disorders. Int J Oral Maxillofac Surg 1993;22:200–9.

[34] Tasaki MM, Westesson PL. Temporomandibular joint: diagnostic accuracy with sagittal and coronal MR imaging. Radiology 1993;186:723–9.

[35] Whyte AM, McNamara D, Rosenberg I, et al. Magnetic resonance imaging in the evaluation of temporomandibular joint disc displacement—a review of 144 cases. Int J Oral Maxillofac Surg 2006;35:696–703.

[36] Tallents RH, Katzberg RW, Murphy W, et al. Magnetic resonance imaging findings in asymptomatic volunteers and symptomatic patients with temporomandibular disorders. J Prosthet Dent 1996;75:529–33.

[37] Tasaki MM, Westesson PL, Raubertas RF. Observer variation in interpretation of magnetic resonance images of the temporomandibular joint. Oral Surg Oral Med Oral Pathol 1993;76: 231–4.

[38] Dolwick MF. Intra-articular disk displacement. Part I: its questionable role in temporomandibular joint pathology. J Oral Maxillofac Surg 1995;53:1069–72.

[39] Coutinho A, Fenyo-Pereira M, Lauria L, et al. The role of SPECT/CT with 99mTc-MDP image fusion to diagnose temporomandibular dysfunction. Oral Surg Oral Med Oral Pathol Oral Radiol Endod 2006;101:224–30.

THE DENTAL
CLINICS
OF NORTH AMERICA

Dent Clin N Am 52 (2008) 891–915

Diagnostic Imaging and Sleep Medicine

Robert A. Strauss, DDS, MD*,
Corey C. Burgoyne, DMD

*Department of Oral and Maxillofacial Surgery, Virginia Commonwealth University Medical
Center, Medical College of Virginia Hospitals, P.O. Box 980566,
Richmond, VA 23298-0566, USA*

Of the approximately 70 million Americans who complain of snoring, an estimated 20%—approximately 15 million people—actually have OSAS. Unfortunately, because of the difficulty in obtaining a proper diagnosis, 80% of the cases remain undiagnosed [1]. Previous data from a cohort study (adults aged 30–60 years) showed the lifetime incidence of OSAS to be 9% to 24% for men and 4% to 9% for women. The estimated prevalence (percent of the population affected at any given time) of OSAS is 4% in men and 2% in women [2]. Similar data have been reported from epidemiologic studies [3].

Risk factors for OSAS include a family history of sleep apnea, a large neck, a recessed chin, any abnormalities in the structure of the upper airway, smoking, alcohol use, and age. In addition to loud snoring and excessive daytime sleepiness, presenting signs and symptoms include high blood pressure and other cardiovascular complications, morning headaches, memory problems, feelings of depression, gastroesophageal reflux, nocturia, and impotence. Excessive weight is a predominant physical characteristic and compounding factor to the prevalence of OSAS. Aside from better recognition, one reason for the increasing number of OSAS diagnoses is the increasing percentage of Americans who are obese. More than 50% of the American population has a body mass index (weight in kg/height in m^2) of more than 30, and research has shown a strong correlation between obesity and nocturnal respiratory disturbance [4]. A large population-based study also showed that the level of disturbance is directly proportional to the degree of obesity [5].

* Corresponding author.
E-mail address: rastraus@vcu.edu (R.A. Strauss).

doi:10.1016/j.cden.2008.06.002 *dental.theclinics.com*

More dentists are getting involved in the diagnosis and management of OSAS. Oral and maxillofacial surgeons are well suited to perform any surgical interventions necessary, from diagnostic nasopharyngoscopy to soft tissue airway procedures (eg, uvulopalatopharyngoplasty, genioglossus muscle advancement, tongue base surgery) to major maxillomandibular advancement telegnathic surgery. General dentists are also becoming more involved, however, specifically in the area of dental appliances to maintain or advance mandibular position during sleep. These appliances have been shown to be as effective as a first-line treatment as the traditional primary treatment method—continuous positive airway pressure [6]. Many people visit their dentist on a more regular basis than their physicians, and dentists have an excellent opportunity to provide screening for the signs and symptoms of OSAS on their health history forms and during the discussion phase of their dental treatment. This screening allows patients to be referred in a timely fashion to an oral and maxillofacial surgeon and formal sleep physician specialist for definitive diagnosis and imaging.

Diagnosis

The initial diagnosis of OSAS is almost always made while taking a good history. Although the history (eg, excessive daytime sleepiness, loud snoring) is a valid screening tool, it is not reliably diagnostic. Up to 30% of patients who have sleep apnea have no signs or symptoms other than loud snoring [7]. Another important assessment tool for the degree of interrupted sleep that a patient experiences is the Epworth Sleepiness Scale, which is a subjective score of a patient's tendency to fall asleep during specific nonstimulating situations, such as driving a car or watching a movie. Although a history and the Epworth Sleepiness Scale can provide some insight into the likelihood that a patient may have OSAS, it is clear that an objective mechanism for diagnosis is necessary before any treatment begins.

The gold standard for diagnosis of OSAS is the polysomnogram (PSG). Polysomnography is a monitored sleep study that is performed in a sleep laboratory and can be performed during the day or night (depending on the patient's normal sleep time) to evaluate a patient during the sleep cycle. The typical PSG has 11 parameters, such as electroencephalogram, monitoring of air flow, electroymogram of the chin, legs, and ocular muscles (also known as electro-oculogram), electrocardiogram, and monitoring of oxygen saturation and chest wall movement. These parameters are evaluated by a sleep specialist and are interpreted in multiple ways to determine the extent of the interrupted sleep experienced by the patient. The report from the PSG provides objective data on the type and frequency of any sleep-related breathing abnormalities, the duration and degree of these abnormalities, and any cardiac, neurologic, or pulmonary consequences of these events (eg, cardiac arrythmias).

Definitions

An OSA event is defined as a cessation of breathing during sleep that lasts for 10 seconds or more, is associated with at least a 2% drop in oxygen saturation, and leads to an arousal from sleep on electroencephalogram (although the definitions vary somewhat by clinical center). Hypopnea is a period of time during which breathing is reduced by at least 50% with a similar decrease in oxygen saturation and arousal. These are laboratory diagnoses. OSAS is defined as having these objective events and having signs and symptoms from these abnormalities, such as daytime somnolence and snoring. The PSG provides objective data in the form of an apnea-hypopnea index, which is the total number of apneic and hypopneic events divided by the number of hours of sleep. Some laboratories also provide a respiratory disturbance index (RDI), which is the total number of apneic and hypopneic events plus the respiratory effort related arousals, which are arousals during sleep that do not meet the strict apneic or hypopneic criteria (eg, lasting less than 10 seconds or not associated with a significant drop in oxygen saturation). A normal apnea-hypopnea index is evidenced by fewer than five events per hour, whereas OSA is defined as more than five apneic or hypopneic events. Depending on the degree of associated desaturation, between 5 and 20 events per hour may be classified as mild to moderate sleep apnea, which can be associated with increased risks such as hypertension, stroke, and cardiac disease. In moderate to severe OSA, when the RDI exceeds 20 (and in some patients may approach 100 events per hour), a dramatic increase in morbidity and mortality may be present [8]. A list of potential physical and mental consequences is shown in Box 1.

Although the PSG provides clinicians with an objective and reproducible mechanism to define the presence and extent of OSAS, it does nothing to elucidate the actual cause or site of the obstruction. Once the diagnosis is made, it is equally important to determine the site and level of the obstruction so that appropriate nonsurgical and surgical treatment planning can be undertaken. OSAS may be caused by obstruction anywhere in the upper airway, from the tip of the nose to the larynx. Many cases of OSAS are caused by obstruction at multiple levels, either simultaneously or in an alternating pattern. Box 2 lists some of the pathologic areas of obstruction. In some cases, however, the problem is not a pathologic entity but excessive mobility of the tissues within the airway, allowing for collapse during inspiration. It is important that the likely cause and site of obstruction be elucidated so that targeted treatment may be instituted.

Imaging

Diagnostic imaging techniques have improved significantly the understanding of the pathophysiology of OSAS. They allow for evaluation and treatment planning of surgical and nonsurgical therapeutic interventions

---

Box 1. Physical and mental consequences of OSAS

Excessive daytime sleepiness
Difficulties with concentration and short-term memory
Depression
Social withdrawal
Nocturnal awakening
Insomnia
Nocturia
Loud snoring
Weight gain
Truncal/visceral obesity
Menopausal status in women
Hypertension
Pulmonary hypertension
Stroke
Insulin resistance
Diabetes mellitus
Serum lipid abnormalities
Serum lipid abnormalities
Elevated C-reactive protein
Elevated liver enzymes

---

that are specific to a patient's likely source of obstruction. Several different imaging tools are currently being used in the diagnosis and treatment planning of OSAS. They range from direct examination using mirror or endoscopic visualization of the nasal and hypopharyngeal airway to sophisticated new techniques, such as three-dimensional MRI and three-dimensional cone beam tomography. It is important to understand that each modality has advantages and disadvantages, and it is up to individual clinicians to decide which imaging technique would best be used for any individual patient.

Panorex

Panoramic radiography (Fig. 1) is commonly used in assessing the hard tissue of the maxilla and mandible in dental offices. Panoramic radiography allows for identification of hard tissue anatomy, such as the location of impacted teeth, the location of the inferior alveolar nerve canal, evaluation of the maxillary sinuses, and the anatomy of the condylar head, all of which may be useful in ruling out anatomic abnormalities that are causing obstruction or, more commonly, any anatomic issues that could affect hard tissue surgical procedures, such as maxillomandibular telegnathic surgery. Little

Box 2. Pathologic conditions associated with OSAS

Nose
Deviated septum
Polyposis
Septal hematoma
Septal dislocation
Rhinitis
Turbinate hypertrophy

Nasopharynx
Carcinoma
Adenoidal hypertrophy
Lymphoma
Choanal stenosis or atresia
Pharyngeal flap
Papillomatosis

Mouth and oropharynx
Hypertrophied tonsils
Elongated and/or thickened palate and uvula
Lymphoma of tonsils, lingual cyst
Lingual tonsillar hypertrophy
Macroglossia: acromegaly
Micrognathia: congenital or acquired
Lipoma of the neck
Hunter syndrome
Hurler syndrome
Head and neck burns
Papillomatosis

Hypopharynx
Floppy or elongated epiglottis
Mass of the valecula
Epiglottic edema
Excessive compliance of the pharyngeal walls

Larynx
Edema of epiglottis
Vocal cord paralysis
Laryngomalacia collapse of aryepiglottic folds

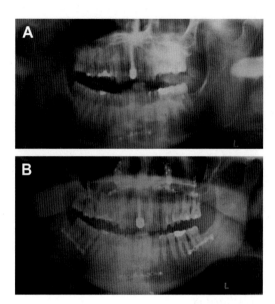

Fig. 1. (*A*, *B*) Preoperative panorex of a patient who underwent bimaxillary advancement surgery.

diagnostic information specific for the diagnosis of OSAS is obtained from the panorex; however, it does provide preoperative documentation of existing anatomy important in the surgical treatment planning, and it provides a postoperative assessment of surgical intervention and anatomic changes.

Rose and colleagues used the panoramic radiograph to monitor the dental condition for patients who have OSAS who were being treated with oral protrusive devices. Healthy oral conditions with sufficient dental retention for the device are essential for successful outcomes using dental appliances for OSAS. They concluded that periodontal disease and unwanted orthodontic movement of the teeth could result from such devices, which limits the indication of this therapeutic approach in some patients. They suggest that to maximize treatment success and minimize dental side effects, close collaboration with dental colleagues and routine panoramic radiographs is necessary in treating patients who have OSAS with an oral protrusive device [9].

Lateral cephalometric radiography

Plain film radiography is the most widely used modality for evaluating the hard and soft tissue anatomy of patients who have OSAS [10]. Lateral cephalometric radiography is used routinely by orthodontists and oral and maxillofacial surgeons for evaluating the facial skeleton. Advantages of lateral cephalometric radiography are that it is inexpensive and minimally invasive, it exposes patients to low-dose radiation (0.005 mSv) [11], and it is easily obtained in the office setting. Standard positioning of the patient during the lateral cephalogram is with the patient's left side toward the film (the patient is facing to his or her left), with Frankfort horizontal (defined as the plane from orbitale to porion) paralleling the horizon, and teeth in centric relation at the end of expiration [12]. The reason for this positioning is that it is a standard, predictable, and reproducible head position that is consistent with the patient's natural head position at rest (Fig. 2).

Many analyses are used to evaluate lateral cephalometric radiographs, predominately for use in orthognathic surgery. Specific measurements for assessing the airway are useful in evaluating patients with OSA [13–15]:

- Soft palate length (PNS-P): the distance from posterior nasal spine (PNS) to the tip of the soft palate
- Posterior airway space (PAS): the distance from the base of the tongue to the posterior pharyngeal wall along the line from B-point through gonion
- Minimum posterior airway space: the narrowest point in the pharynx
- Mandibular plane to hyoid distance (MP-H): the distance determined by measuring a perpendicular line from the mandibular plane to the hyoid bone
- Bony nasopharynx (PNS-Ba): PNS to basion
- Bony oropharynx (PNS-AA): PNS to anterior border of the atlas (C2)
- Tonsillar size (T): perpendicular distance at the maximum convexity of the tonsil
- Tonsillar pharyngeal ratio (TP): the ratio of the width of the tonsil (T) to the depth of the pharyngeal space (PAS).

Patients who have OSAS have abnormal cephalometric anatomy, which may be a function of the hard and/or the soft tissue (Figs. 3 and 4) [14,16,17].

Yu and Fujimoto and colleagues examined the radiographic findings of 62 obese and nonobese patients who have OSAS. Their data showed that

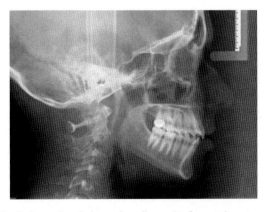

Fig. 2. Lateral cephalometric radiograph of normal anatomy.

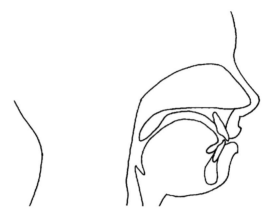

Fig. 3. Line drawing of airway anatomy.

patients who have OSAS consistently have upper airway narrowing at the soft palate (short minimum posterior airway space), a longer soft palate (long PNS-P), an inferiorly positioned hyoid bone (long MP-H), narrowing of the bony nasopharynx (shorter PNS-Ba), and narrowing of the bony oropharynx (shorter PNS-AA). In comparing the obese patient and nonobese patients, the soft tissue differences were much more significant in obese patients [14], which indicated that adipose deposition in the upper airway may aggravate the severity of OSAS.

Because patients who have OSAS have abnormal cephalometric anatomy, researchers have studied whether the cephalometric measures may indicate a higher risk for severity of OSAS disease. Partinen and colleagues evaluated 157 patients who have OSAS by obtaining lateral cephalometric radiographs and PSG data. The results showed two important correlations: (1) that patients with OSAS consistently have longer mandibular plane to

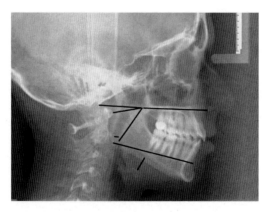

Fig. 4. Linear measurements used in airway assessment.

hyoid distance (MP-H) and more narrow posterior airway space (PAS), and (2) that when MP-H distance is more than 24 mm and PAS width is 5 mm or less, the RDI, as determined by the polysomnogram, is elevated. This study indicated that the severity of a low hyoid and a narrow posterior airway space is consistent with a higher risk for elevated RDI. Naganuma and colleagues obtained cephalometric and endoscopic studies on 64 patients previously diagnosed with OSAS or snoring. Statistically significant correlations were found between the apnea hypopnea index and minimum posterior airway space and mandibular plane to hyoid (MP-H) distance. The apnea hypopnea index increased with a minimum posterior airway space distance of less than 7 mm and an MP-H distance of more than 27.4 mm [16].

When assessing patients who have OSAS, it is important to distinguish between adult and the pediatric patients. OSAS is becoming a more frequently diagnosed disease in children, and studies have found the prevalence to be 2% to 4% in the US population [18]. Similar to adults, there are many physiologic causes for OSAS in children, yet one significant difference is that adenotonsillar hypertrophy is the most common cause of OSAS in children [19]. Li and Wong and colleagues [14] measured TP ratio on standard lateral cephalometric radiographs and performed overnight PSG in 35 children. The tonsillar size is determined by measuring the perpendicular distance at the maximum convexity of the tonsil (Fig. 5). The TP ratio is the tonsillar width (T) divided by the pharyngeal depth (PAS). All children in the study had some degree of tonsillar hypertrophy, and the TP ratio ranged from 0.65 to 0.8, meaning that on average the pediatric airways were 65% to 80% occluded by the tonsils. A significant correlation was found between the TP ratio and the RDI, which indicated a positive relationship between the amount of airway occlusion by the tonsils and the severity of OSAS [15].

Plain film lateral cephalometric radiographs have excellent application in the assessment of patients who have OSAS. Lateral cephalometric

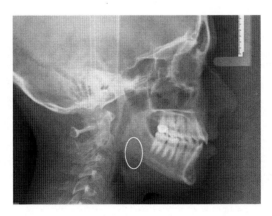

Fig. 5. Representation of the tonsillar assessment on a lateral cephalometric radiograph.

radiographs are widely available, easily obtained and reproducible, inexpensive, noninvasive, and useful in evaluation the bony and soft tissue anatomy that contributes to OSAS, and they require minimal radiation exposure. The limitations of the lateral cephalometric radiograph are that it is a static, two-dimensional image that is obtained with the patient in the upright position. This is significant because the lateral cephalogram does not represent the airway anatomy in the same position as it is during an apneic event. Variations in the measurement and interpretation of cephalometric data are weaknesses of these studies as are the questionable correlations with anatomic differences and severity of disease.

Independently, cephalometric imaging is not a panacea for the diagnosis of patients who have OSAS. It is the author's view that the lateral cephalometric radiograph is an excellent screening tool and resource for evaluation, treatment planning, and postoperative assessment (Fig. 6) of patients who have OSA because of its ability to delineate two-dimensional anatomy, show excellent hard tissue structures, and be obtained in the general practitioner's office with minimal cost and radiation exposure to the patient. It is also the author's recommendations to assess cephalometric data in light of the polysomnogram, clinical history, and physical examination.

CT

CT is a high-resolution radiographic examination of the hard and soft tissue of the head and neck. When compared with lateral cephalometric radiographs, CT scanning offers greater anatomic detail in three dimensions. A standard CT image is obtained as a single point in time represented by serial two-dimensional images in either a coronal or axial view. The data from the serial two-dimensional images can be interpreted by a computer and be reformatted into a three-dimensional image. CT scanning is discussed in this article as standard CT imaging, fast CT, and cone beam imaging (Fig. 7).

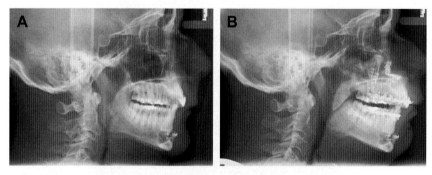

Fig. 6. (*A*) Preoperative and (*B*) postoperative lateral cephalometric radiograph of a patient who underwent bimaxillary advancement surgery.

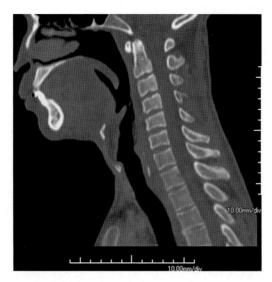

Fig. 7. Standard neck CT shown in a sagittal, bony window.

Standard CT imaging

The standard CT of the head and neck is subdivided into four standard studies: the cranium, maxilla, mandible, and neck. The images are obtained as 1- to 2-mm slices in axial or coronal planes or both. These slices can be combined to obtain a high-resolution three-dimensional image useful in assessing hard and soft tissue of the entire airway from the nares to the hypopharynx. The CT scan provides not only two- and three-dimensional images of the airway anatomy but also a volumetric analysis of the airway. When assessing a patient who has OSAS, this view of the entire airway is essential because the pathophysiology of OSAS can occur anywhere in the upper airway.

Li and colleagues [20] studied 194 patients who have sleep-disordered breathing with standard CT scanning to evaluate the lateral and anteroposterior dimensions of the retropalatal and the retroglossal spaces in patients who have OSAS. They compared the anatomic values to the RDI and showed that the smaller the retropalatal dimension, the higher the RDI. Their results showed that the lateral dimension of the retropalatal space is the anatomic feature most strongly correlated with the severity of the RDI.

Another study by Yucel and colleagues [21] evaluated 47 patients who have OSAS by obtaining CT images during various phases of respiration. Their data showed that patients who have severe OSAS have a significantly narrower cross-sectional area at the level of the uvula, an inferiorly positioned hyoid bone, and a thicker soft palate. These studies support the anatomic variations that exist in patients who have OSAS, suggesting that airway obstruction likely occurs at the level of the palate and the base of tongue.

Standard CT scans are high resolution, provide two- and three-dimensional and volumetric analysis of the airway, are obtained in the supine position, are minimally invasive, and are accessible at most hospital facilities. Shortcomings of the CT scan are the increased cost, radiation exposure to the patient (0.2–1.0 rad/1.5 mSv) [22], static image, and poorer quality imaging of soft tissue. CT imaging is a useful and accessible diagnostic tool for providing images with high resolution and in multiple dimensions, but the cost and inconvenience make this study less practical on a routine basis.

Fast CT imaging

Because sleep apnea is a physiologic disease associated with the dynamic movement of hard and soft tissues, capturing the dynamic nature of the tissue is important in assessing patients who have OSAS. The time component of sleep apnea can be assessed by fast CT, which is a rapid CT scan that allows for acquisition of eight contiguous scans every 0.7 seconds. This rapid imaging provides the dynamic assessment of the upper airway during different stages of the respiratory cycle. Fast CT, like standard CT, obtains two-dimensional images that can be reconstructed to provide a three-dimensional image. CT technology has been able to show that airway compliance (a percentage change in the area of the airway during the respiratory cycle) plays a significant role in contributing to airway obstruction.

Lan and colleagues [22] obtained fast CT scans for the evaluation of patients who have OSAS. The airway was assessed in awake and asleep patients using computer software to determine the volume and compliance of the pharyngeal airway. Their results showed that patients who have OSAS have a relatively higher pharyngeal compliance. This increase in compliance is a result of decreased muscle tonus or increased soft tissue mass or both. This increase in compliance occurs at the middle and hypopharynx, whereas the velopharynx (area between the soft palate and the posterior pharyngeal wall) is the smallest area in caliber of the entire pharyngeal airway. Lan and colleagues [23] concluded that narrowing or collapse of the upper pharynx is caused by the smaller baseline caliber alone and that the collapse of the middle pharynx is the result of higher compliance and small caliber.

The fast CT provides a more physiologically significant assessment of the upper airway compared with standard CT imaging because of its ability to capture the dynamic component of sleep apnea. It carries the same drawbacks of standard CT imaging because of increased cost, radiation exposure to the patient, and inconvenience of obtaining the image.

Cone beam imaging

Cone beam imaging is becoming a popular imaging modality in dentistry and dental specialties. Cone beam imaging uses low-dose radiation to obtain a standard image format that can be manipulated on various computer platforms in two and three dimensions (Fig. 8).

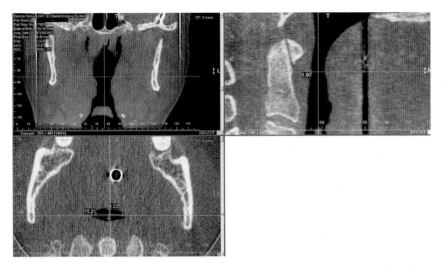

Fig. 8. Cone beam image shows the ability to measure airway parameters in three dimensions. (*Courtesy of* Steven Guttenberg, DDS, MD, Washington, DC).

Mischkowski and colleagues [24] compared the accuracy of cone beam imaging units to standard CT imaging by examining radiopaque markers on dry human skulls. They assessed the accuracy of linear and volumetric measurements, and their results indicated that the evaluated cone beam device provides satisfactory information about linear distances and volumes. Standard CT scans proved slightly more accurate in both measurement categories, but the difference is not relevant for most clinical applications. Ogawa and colleagues [25] evaluated 20 patients with and without OSAS using cone beam tomography to compare their upper airway structure. Information gathered from the cone beam images included the location and shape of the smallest cross-sectional area of the pharyngeal airway, the anteroposterior and lateral dimensions of the airway, and the length of the soft palate. In comparison to patients who do not have OSA, patients who have OSA showed significant constriction of the pharyngeal airway, particularly in the anteroposterior dimension, with the smallest cross-sectional area occurring below the occlusal plane, giving the airway an elliptic configuration.

Cone beam imaging is widely available and is becoming a more highly used imaging modality in dental and dental specialties, which makes it more accessible and practical for routine use. The cone beam device is a compact, office-sized machine that is relatively less expensive than standard CT imaging, and it exposes patients to comparatively low-dose radiation, which is specific to each manufacturer and design. The image can be obtained in sitting and supine positions with accurate assessment of the upper airway cross-sectional area and volume, with excellent bony anatomy, and three-dimensional reconstruction capability. The main disadvantages of cone beam imaging are initial cost, static image, and poor soft tissue resolution. At the time of this writing, there is limited literature on cone beam imaging in evaluating patients who have OSAS, so as this imaging modality becomes more widely used there may be further implications in its use.

MRI

MRI is an imaging modality that is commonly used in the assessment of soft tissue. MRI uses electromagnetic energy and radio waves to assess various soft tissue types without exposing a patient to ionizing radiation. MR images can be obtained in any plane, in comparison to standard CT, which is predominately taken in the axial and coronal planes. MRI has equal resolution but much greater soft tissue contrast than CT scanning, which allows more detailed visualization of soft tissues. In particular, MRI provides an excellent image for examining the soft tissue of the airway (Fig. 9).

Schotland and colleagues [26] used MRI to assess upper airway musculature (genioglossus, geniohyoid, sternohyoid, sternothyroid) in patients who have OSAS. They found that the suprahyoid muscles (genioglossus and geniohyoid) differed between the apneic and control groups, whereas infrahyoid (sternohyoid and sternothyroid) muscles were similar between groups. Comparing OSAS and control groups showed increased soft tissue (edema

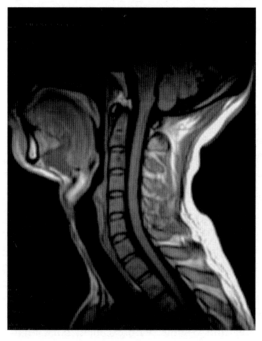

Fig. 9. Standard neck MRI in a sagittal window.

and fat) content of the tongue muscles in patients who have OSAS, but there was little difference between the infrahyoid muscles. Schwab and Goldberg [27] used volumetric analysis and MRI to assess the anatomic soft tissue risk factors for sleep-disordered breathing. They showed that the volume of upper airway soft tissue structures is enlarged in patients who have OSA. The enlargement of these structures represents a significant risk factor for sleep apnea, and the tongue and lateral wall volumes are particularly important independent risk factors for sleep apnea.

Rapid image acquisition MRI can be used to examine the airway in a dynamic fashion. By obtaining rapid images that are temporally spaced a short time apart, a computer can collate the images and play them back in a movie-like fashion. Fast MRI can obtain 0.8 images at 1 image per 1 second, which allows not only multidimensional views but also visualization of the changing shape and configuration of the airway during inspiration and expiration. Ciscar and colleagues [28] used fast MRI to assess the airway of patients who have OSAS and showed they have a smaller velopharynx, a greater variation in velopharyngeal diameter between awake and asleep states, and larger palatal and pharyngeal fat pads. They concluded that the changes in the velopharynx area and diameter during the respiratory cycle are greater in patients who have OSAS, particularly during sleep. This finding suggests that patients who have OSAS have a more collapsible velopharynx, which is the main cause of airway obstruction.

Schoenberg and colleagues [29] studied obstructive pharyngeal changes in sleeping patients who have OSAS by dynamic MRI and concurrent electroencephalogram monitoring. They showed complete airway collapse during apneic events, which occurred at the level of the soft palate and base of tongue. They compared the apneic event to a Mueller's maneuver (discussed later in this article in the section on diagnostic nasopharyngoscopy) and found that there was neither the same extent of pharyngeal narrowing nor a complete collapse of the airway during the Mueller's maneuver as in the apneic event seen on MRI. The process of MRI is loud; patients were sleep deprived before the study, and special precautions were taken to stifle the noise of the MRI machine to enhance the study. The time with which it takes to obtain an MRI and the loud noise of the machine itself were clearly drawbacks of MRI imaging in vivo. The significance of this study, however, was that Schoenberg and colleagues [29] were able to correlate the true apneic event with an image of the airway soft tissue anatomy during the event.

MRI provides an image with excellent contrast of the soft tissue anatomy associated with OSAS. The use of dynamic MRI is important because of its ability to capture the airway anatomy at the time of the apneic event. Other benefits of MRI are that it does not expose patients to ionizing radiation and it allows for imaging to be obtained in multiple planes. The major limitations of MRI are that the machine is large, the scanner is noisy, obtaining the image normally takes several minutes (unless using fast MRI), many people experience claustrophobic effects while in the gantry tube, and it is expensive. The lack of a comfortable sleep environment also limits the ability to use MRI during sleep.

Although standard MRI shows anatomic variation between patients with and without OSAS and although the fast MRI is able to show the anatomic obstruction dynamically during apnea, the cost, inconvenience, and limited availability negate the use of MRI as a routine imaging assessment for patients who have OSAS. This imaging modality may be reserved for more complicated and recalcitrant cases. These images are not necessary for diagnosis; however, they can be helpful in deciding how to treat patients who have OSA. As the cost and other detrimental factors of using MRI diminish, the advantage of this nonionizing radiation modality will increase its use in the future.

Nasopharyngoscopy

Nasopharyngoscopy involves the use of a flexible fiberoptic endoscope passed through the nasal cavity into the pharynx that provides for direct examination of the caliber of the upper airway. It allows the surgeon who is contemplating surgery to rule out any other pathologic sources of obstruction in the airway, such as nasal polyps, vocal cord lesions or paralysis, or tongue base neoplasm. This examination is mandatory before performing airway surgery or any other type of intervention for OSAS. When used in conjunction with a Mueller's maneuver (forced inspiration against a closed airway to mimic airway closure during an apneic event), nasopharyngoscopy may be useful in diagnosing the level of obstruction in OSAS. The ability to see the airway directly, in real-time, and in all dimensions makes this an attractive alternative to radiologic and other indirect imaging modalities.

To perform diagnostic nasal endoscopy, the only equipment required is the scope itself, a light source, and some topical anesthesia mixed with a decongestant or vasoconstrictor (eg, lidocaine or pontocaine mixed with oxymetazole or neosynephrine). A video camera can involve the patient and the office staff while making visibility easier for the surgeon, but this also increases the cost of the equipment (Fig. 10) [30].

Nasopharyngoscopy is performed with the patient initially in an upright position and is generally tolerated with minimal discomfort after application of topical anesthesia to the patient's nose and palate. A 3- to 5-mm flexible nasopharyngoscope is inserted into the anterior chamber and the middle meatus of the nose to assess for turbinate hypertrophy or septal deviation. The scope is advanced forward within the inferior meatus using gentle pressure to examine the nasopharynx and eustachian tubes as potential areas of obstruction. The palate is identified, and the patient is placed in the horizontal position and asked to perform a Mueller maneuver (taking a deep breath through closed nostrils with a closed mouth, thereby generating negative intrapharyngeal pressures). The estimated percent of airway collapse at

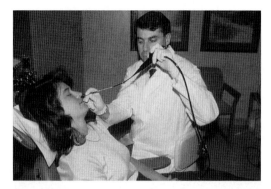

Fig. 10. Example of nasopharyngoscope being passed into airway. Note that the procedure can be done with the surgeon either sitting or standing. The patient can be in the sitting position or the reclining position.

the level of the nasopharynx is recorded at maximal inspiration (Fig. 11). The scope subsequently is advanced to the oropharynx, where the base of the tongue is inspected as a possible area of obstruction. The scope is advanced to the hypopharynx, where specific attention is turned to the lateral pharyngeal walls and another Mueller maneuver is performed to assess for retroglossal collapse (Figs. 12 and 13). This is followed by an evaluation of the patient's larynx. After removal of the scope, the opposite nasal passage is inspected. Although this maneuver would seem to mimic airway collapse and some studies show a clear correlation with the finding on Mueller's maneuver and the effectiveness of particular procedures that correct abnormalities in a specific portion of the airway, other studies have

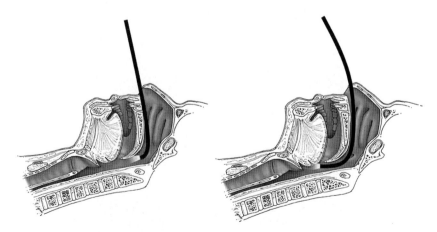

Fig. 11. Diagramming the placement of the scope into the nasopharynx and oropharynx. (*From* Strauss RA. Flexible endoscopic nasopharyngoscopy. Atlas of the Oral and Maxillofacial Surgery Clinics 2007;15(2):111–28; with permission.)

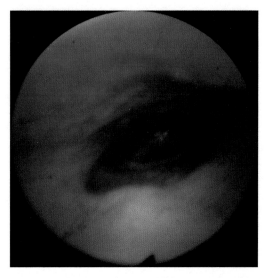

Fig. 12. Muller's maneuver at level of soft palate before the maneuver. Note the wide open airway.

found no such correlation. The use of the maneuver for definitive treatment planning has to be considered carefully.

The Fujita classification of the upper airway, often used to identify the area of obstruction in patients who have OSAS, is based on nasopharyngoscopy findings. In type I, the area of obstruction is considered to be

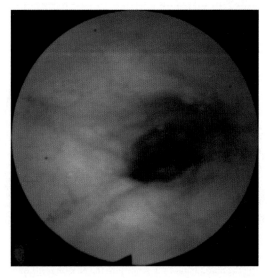

Fig. 13. Muller's maneuver at level of soft palate during the maneuver. Note the approximate 50% decrease in airway size.

oropharyngeal and is solely retropalatal. In type II, the area of obstruction is between the oropharynx and hypopharynx; it is classified further into type IIa, which is a more retropalatal obstruction, and type IIb, which is a more retroglossal obstruction. In type III, the area of obstruction is confined to the hypopharynx and is solely retroglossal. There is much debate in the literature about the accuracy of nasopharyngoscopy in determining the level of obstruction because obstruction probably moves from place to place within the airway, occurs at multiple levels simultaneously, and is more likely during sleep than during wakefulness (as when the nasopharyngoscopy is performed). Some evidence in the literature indicates that performing nasopharygoscopy with the patient sedated may increase the reliability of detecting sleep related obstruction, but this also carries with it the risk of parenteral sedation in a sleep apnea patient—a significant risk given the compromise of the airway inherent in this disease.

Diagnostic nasopharyngoscopy is an in-office, simple, easy, and painless method for physically imaging the upper airway directly and provides real-time data on possible sources and levels of obstruction. It is easy to learn and inexpensive to perform. The limitation of an awake patient and questionable correlation to sleep-related obstruction should caution the surgeon to use these data as one more piece of a complex puzzle, and its findings should be added and correlated to the findings other imaging and diagnostic tests before treatment planning.

Acoustic reflection

Acoustic reflection is a minimally invasive technique that uses sound waves reflected into the upper airway to provide a physical image of the airway and pharyngeal airflow. It can be useful for measuring upper airway obstruction. An acoustic probe is inserted into the mouth and generates an audible sound signal, which is transmitted through the mouth into the oropharynx and hypopharynx (Fig. 14). The acoustic wave changes when it encounters impedance (resistance to airflow) [31] and is reflected back to a microphone or a semiconductor pressure transducer in the wave tube. The change in amplitude of the sound as it passes through the upper airway is measured by a computer that subsequently calculates the cross-sectional area of the airway.

Gelardi and colleagues [32] compared 110 patients with and without OSAS by using acoustic pharyngometry to assess the upper airway. Their results showed a significant increase in airway resistance in patients who have OSAS, and they concluded that acoustic pharyngometry was a useful method in determining the diagnosis and assessing the severity of obstructive sleep apnea.

A benefit of acoustic reflection is that it is a minimally invasive study that does not require exposure to radiation. It provides a dynamic assessment of the airway, and it is easily repeatable. Downfalls of acoustic reflection are

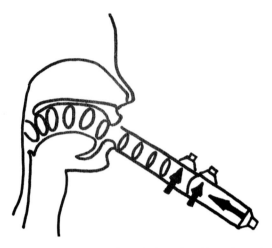

Fig. 14. Diagram of the acoustic probe introduced into the oral cavity.

that it is generally performed in the sitting position, it does not provide an anatomic representation of the airway, and it is performed through the mouth, which alters the upper airway anatomy. Unlike other modalities that are passive, this is an active process that requires input by the patient, thereby precluding performing the procedure in a sedated patient, which might be more accurate than doing the test in an awake patient. Acoustic pharyngometry is an adjunctive method of evaluating the airway, but the lack of literature validating this technique indicates that acoustic pharyngometry currently provides little information about the anatomy or disease status in patients who have OSAS.

Fluoroscopy

Fluoroscopy is an imaging modality that uses a continuous x-ray beam against a mobile fluorescent plate to obtain dynamic images of internal structures of a patient. Fluoroscopy is commonly used for evaluating the gastrointestinal tract and for angiography (in which it can be used to allow immediate visualization during intravenous infusions of radiographic dye) and for orthopedic surgery (in which it allows for intraoperative assessment of fracture alignment). Because of its dynamic real-time visualization, it also may be useful for assessing the fluid nature of the hard and soft tissue anatomy of the upper airway during inspiration. Pepin and colleagues [33] combined standard fluoroscopy with polysomnography (somnofluoroscopy) to evaluate the upper airway during sleep studies. They were able to correlate specific anatomic fluoroscopic changes in the upper airway with apneic events. Yoshida and colleagues [34] conducted a similar study by using low-field fluoroscopy to assess the upper airway status of 20 patients who have OSAS. The patients were imaged for 5 minutes while awake and

30 minutes while asleep; 19 of the 20 patients did not require any sedative drugs to induce sleep because of the lack of noise created by the fluoroscopy unit. None of the patients showed obstruction while awake, but during sleep, all 20 patients showed some degree of obstruction at the retropalatal pharynx. They concluded that airway closure occurs in the retropalatal region and that fluoroscopy is a useful diagnostic study to examine upper airway obstruction in patients who have OSAS [34].

Fluoroscopy not only provides a dynamic view of the upper airway during sleep but also allows for the visualization of anatomic movement outside of the pharyngeal airway. For instance, movements of the cervical spine, downward motion of the hyoid bone, and jaw movements at the end of an apnea can be observed directly. Fluoroscopy also can be performed in the supine position, is minimally invasive, and can avoid the use of sedation anesthesia for achieving a sleep state.

Fluoroscopy has the disadvantage that even when using low-dose radiation, the length of a typical procedure often results in a relatively high absorbed dose to the patient. Fluoroscopy can only visualize the airway in two dimensions, making it difficult to obtain precise measurements of the three-dimensional airway lumen [12]. The ability to visualize the airway anatomy as a dynamic image during sleep is an excellent benefit to the fluoroscopic examination; however, the two-dimensional image, inconvenience, and radiation exposure limit the use of this for the routine assessment of patients who have OSAS.

Manometry

Manometry is the use of catheter probes placed in the pharyngeal airway to detect pressure at various sites in the airway. Manometry is used to identify patients who have sleep disturbances caused by increased airway pressure not indicated by standard polysomnogram measurements. An advantage of using catheter manometry is the ability to obtain airway pressures during an entire night of sleep. Reda and colleagues [35] evaluated 59 snoring patients by overnight polysomnography and simultaneous pharyngoesophageal manometry. Their data showed that manometry was 100% sensitive and specific in excluding OSAS and identifying severe OSAS. The study was not able to distinguish between apnea and hypopneas by the pressure catheters alone, however.

Other authors suggested that manometry provides a poor predictive value for the location of obstruction. The negative inspiratory pressure dissipates in areas superior to the level of the obstruction, making pressure measurements in these areas less accurate. They also concluded that the use of catheters does not provide volumetric data or identify the anatomic structures that contribute to airway collapse and obstruction [36–38].

Manometry is useful in diagnosing increased airway resistance and distinguishing between patients who have severe OSAS and those who do not.

The study can be obtained overnight and at home. The data obtained from pressure catheters are controversial because of the transnasal position and interference of the catheter normal airway function. Manometry is an adjunctive assessment of airway resistance, but it is otherwise less diagnostic than other similarly invasive studies.

Procedural sedation

Most diagnostic imaging of the airway for OSAS is performed with patients awake. This may lead to inaccuracies because the dynamics of the airway are likely different when patients are awake than when they are asleep, which is precisely when OSAS occurs. This is probably caused by the differences in muscular tonus within the airway dilating muscles between these two states. It is ideal to perform any imaging while patients are asleep.

Sedation is commonly used to induce sleep in patients undergoing various modes of diagnostic imaging. Because of the uncomfortable or intimidating situation created by diagnostic imaging, it is difficult to achieve a natural state of sleep necessary to evaluate apnea without induced sedation. Airway compromise is a significant concern in any sedated patient especially in the sleep apnea population because OSAS has been associated with increased perioperative morbidity and mortality [39]. Donnelly and colleagues [40] studied the effects and safety of sedation on 80 children with known airway compromise undergoing fluoroscopy for the assessment of OSAS. They monitored the children for oxygen desaturation and labored breathing and found that none of the children required tracheal intubation, developed respiratory distress requiring the aid of other physicians, or required hospitalization related to sedation for the dynamic sleep fluoroscopy study. They concluded that children with airway compromise who are being evaluated for OSA can be sedated successfully and safely for dynamic sleep fluoroscopy when a structured sedation program is used, including a separate anesthesia provider [40].

Literature concerning adult patients who have OSAS undergoing moderate and deep sedation for diagnostic imaging is lacking. Perioperative studies in patients who have OSAS indicate that these patients are at higher risk for difficult airway management, apnea, increased oxygen requirement, pain-sedation mismatch, and episodes of desaturation [39]. Common side effects of sedative medications are muscle relaxation, respiratory depression, and obtunded reflexes, all of which can exacerbate the apneic events in a patient who has OSAS. Sedation is useful for inducing sleep and evaluating intermittent airway obstruction, but sedation should be used with caution in adults with a known difficult airway. Kheterpal and colleagues assessed the difficulty of mask ventilation and intubation of 22,660 patients and found that 2% of the attempts were either inadequate or unstable, required two providers, or impossible to mask ventilate. They concluded that abnormal neck anatomy, sleep apnea, snoring, and body mass index of 30 kg/m or more were independent predictors of inadequate mask ventilation and difficult intubation [41].

Sedation is a valuable adjunct to diagnostic imaging because it can provide a pharmacologically induced state of sleep. This should likely lead to increased accuracy of diagnostic imaging; however, proper airway skills and vigilance are important when using sedation in adult patients who have OSAS.

Summary

Imaging techniques have provided tremendous advances in the diagnosis, treatment planning, and surgical assessment of the upper airway in patients who have OSAS [27]. There are benefits and limitations to each of the diagnostic imaging techniques for OSAS. Each imaging modality provides a piece of information that, when combined with other data, can be used to determine the severity to the disease and the location of the obstruction and indicate areas of interest for surgical intervention. As imaging techniques continue to progress, the ability to identify the location or cause of the airway obstruction during a true apneic event will continue to improve. Ultimately, the diagnostic study should provide anatomic imaging consistent with the physiologic location and severity of disease with minimal invasion, minimal need for sedation, and limited radiation exposure. OSAS is being diagnosed more readily today because of the multitude of assessment techniques, and the use of diagnostic imaging will continue to be an essential component of the management of the disease.

References

[1] Punjabi NM. The epidemiology of adult obstructive sleep apnea. Proc Am Thorac Soc 2008 Feb;5(2):136–43.

[2] Koo BB, Dostal J, Ioachimescu O, et al. The effects of gender and age on REM-related sleep-disordered breathing. Sleep Breath 2007;12(3):259–64.

[3] Bixler EO, Vgontzas AN, Lin HM, et al. Prevalence of sleep-disordered breathing in women: effects of gender. Am J Respir Crit Care Med 2001;163(3 Pt 1):608–13.

[4] Nieto FJ, Young TB, Lind BK, et al. For the Sleep Heart Health Study Association. Sleep-disordered breathing, sleep apnea, and hypertension in a large community-based study. JAMA 2000;283:1829–36.

[5] Zwillich CW. Is untreated sleep apnea a contributing factor for chronic hypertension? JAMA 2000;283:1880–1.

[6] Ferguson K, Cartwright R, Rogers R. Oral appliances for snoring and obstructive sleep apnea: a review. Sleep 2006;29(2):244–62.

[7] Duran J, Esnaola S, Rubio R, et al. Obstructive sleep apnea-hypopnea and related clinical features in a population based sample of subjects aged 30–70 years. Am J Respir Crit Care Med 2001;163:685–9.

[8] Rundell OH, Jones RK. Polysomnography methods and interpretations. Otolaryngol Clin North Am 1990;23:583–91.

[9] Rose E, Ridder GJ, Staats R, et al. Intraoral protrusion devices in obstructive sleep apnea: dental findings and possible treatments. HNO 2002;50(1):29–34.

[10] Thakkar K, Yao M. Diagnostic studies in obstructive sleep apnea. Otolaryngol Clin North Am 2007;40:785–805.

[11] Ngan DC, Kharbanda OP, Geenty JP, et al. Comparison of radiation levels from computed tomography and conventional dental radiographs. Aust Orthod J 2003;19(2):67–75.

[12] Rama AN, Tekwani SH, Kushida CA. Sites of obstruction in obstructive sleep apnea. Chest 2002;122:1139–47.

[13] Acebo C, Millman RP, Rosenberg C, et al. Sleep, breathing, and cephalometrics in older children and young adults. Chest 1996;109(3):664–72.

[14] Yu X, Fujimoto K, Urushibata K, et al. Cephalometric analysis in obese and nonobese patients with obstructive sleep apnea syndrome. Chest 2003;124(1):212–8.

[15] Li AM, Wong E, Kew J, et al. Use of tonsil size in the evaluation of obstructive sleep apnoea. Arch Dis Child 2002;87:156–9.

[16] Naganuma H, Okamoto M, Woodson BT, et al. Cephalometric and fiberoptic evaluation as a case-selection technique for obstructive sleep apnea syndrome (OSAS). Acta Otolaryngol 2002;547:57–63.

[17] Guilleminault C, Riley R, Powell N. Obstructive sleep apnea and abnormal cephalometric measurements: implications for treatment. Chest 1984;86(5):793–4.

[18] Ali NJ, Pitson D, Stradling JR. The prevalence of snoring, sleep disturbance and sleep related breathing disorders and their relation to daytime sleepiness in 4-5 year old children. Arch Dis Child 1993;68:360–6.

[19] Brouillette RT, Fernbach SK, Hunt CE. Obstructive sleep apnea in infants and children. J Pediatr 1982;100:31–40.

[20] Li HY, Chen NH, Wang CR, et al. Use of 3-dimensional computed tomography scan to evaluate upper airway patency for patients undergoing sleep disordered breathing surgery. Otolaryngol Head Neck Surg 2003;129:336–42.

[21] Yucel A, Unlu M, Haktanir A, et al. Evaluation of the upper airway cross-sectional area changes in different degrees of severity of obstructive sleep apnea syndrome: cephalometric and dynamic CT study. AJNR Am J Neuroradiol 2005;26:2624–9.

[22] Shrimpton PC, Miller HC, Lewis MA, et al. National survey of doses from CT in the UK. 2003. Br J Radiol 2006;79:968–80.

[23] Lan Z, Itoi A, Takashima M, et al. Difference of pharyngeal morphology and mechanical property between OSAHS patients and normal subjects. Auris Nasus Larynx 2006;33: 433–9.

[24] Mischkowski RA, Pulsfort R, Ritter L, et al. Geometric accuracy of a newly developed cone-beam device for maxillofacial imaging. Oral Surg Oral Med Oral Pathol Oral Radiol Endod 2007;104(4):551–9.

[25] Ogawa R, Enciso R, Shintaku W, et al. Evaluation of cross-section airway configuration of obstructive sleep apnea. Oral Surg Oral Med Oral Pathol Oral Radiol Endod 2007;103: 102–8.

[26] Schotland HM, Insko EK, Schwab RJ. Quantitative magnetic resonance imaging demonstrates alterations of the lingual musculature in obstructive sleep apnea. Sleep 1999;22(5): 605–13.

[27] Schwab R, Goldberg A. Upper airway assesment: radiographic and other imaging techniques. Otolaryngol Clin North Am 1998;31(6):931–68.

[28] Ciscar MA, Juan G, Martínez V, et al. Magnetic resonance imaging of the pharynx in OSA patients and healthy subjects. Eur J Respir Dis 2001;17:79–86.

[29] Schoenberg SO, Floemer F, Kroeger H, et al. Combined assessment of obstructive sleep apnea syndrome with dynamic MRI and parallel EEG registration: initial results. Invest Radiol 2000;35(4):267–76.

[30] Strauss RA. Flexible diagnostic nasopharyngoscopy. Atlas Oral Maxillofac Surg Clin North Am 2007;15(2):111–28.

[31] Kamal I. Test-retest validity of acoustic pharyngometry measurements. Otolaryngol Head Neck Surg 2004;130:223–8.

[32] Gelardi M, Del Giudice AM, Cariti F, et al. Acoustic pharyngometry: clinical and instrumental correlations in sleep disorders. Rev Bras Otorrinolaringol (Engl Ed) 2007;73(2): 257–65.
[33] Pepin JL, Ferretti G, Veale D, et al. Somnofluoroscopy, computed tomography, and cephalometry in the assessment of the airway in obstructive sleep apnoea. Thorax 1992;47:150–6.
[34] Yoshida K, Fukatsu H, Ando Y, et al. Evaluation of sleep apnea syndrome with low-field magnetic resonance fluoroscopy. Eur Radiol 1999;9(6):1197–202.
[35] Reda M, Gibson GJ, Wilson JA. Pharyngoesophageal pressure monitoring in sleep apnea syndrome. Otolaryngol Head Neck Surg 2001;125(4):324–31.
[36] Chaban R, Cole P, Hoffstein V. Site of upper airway obstruction in patients with idiopathic obstructive sleep apnea. Laryngoscope 1988;98:641–7.
[37] Woodson ET, Wooten MR. A multisensor solid-state pressure manometer to identify the level of collapse in obstructive sleep apnea. Otolaryngol Head Neck Surg 1992;107:651–6.
[38] Hudgel DW, Harasick T, Katz RL, et al. Uvulopalatopharyngoplasty in obstructive apnea: value of preoperative localization of site of upper airway narrowing during sleep. Am Rev Respir Dis 1991;143:942–6.
[39] Gali B, Whalen FX Jr, Gay PC, et al. Management plan to reduce risks in perioperative care of patients with presumed obstructive sleep apnea syndrome. J Clin Sleep Med 2007;3(6): 582–8.
[40] Donnelly LF, Strife JL, Myer CM III. Is sedation safe during dynamic sleep fluoroscopy of children with obstructive sleep apnea? AJR Am J Roentgenol 2001;177(5):1031–4.
[41] Kheterpal S, Han R, Tremper KK, et al. Incidence and predictors of difficult and impossible mask ventilation. Anesthesiology 2006;105(5):885–91.

THE DENTAL
CLINICS
OF NORTH AMERICA

ELSEVIER
SAUNDERS

Dent Clin N Am 52 (2008) 917–928

The Future of Dental and Maxillofacial Imaging

Dale A. Miles, DDS, MS, FRCD(C)[a,b,*]

[a]*University of Texas at San Antonio, San Antonio, TX, USA*
[b]*Arizona School of Dentistry and Oral Health, Mesa TX, USA*

This issue of *Dental Clinics of North America* has covered old and new imaging modalities, their current applications, and some more contemporary applications such as image-guided surgery. What is left to be said?

I will start first with what dentists and oral and maxillofacial radiologists will most likely not do, even with our newest imaging technique—cone beam volumetric tomography (CBVT).

Although at least one manufacturer has previously shown vessels in the head and neck region in their CBVT machine brochure, dentists and oral radiologists will probably never do contrast procedures. Blood is not stationary, and to see the flow patterns, contrast nonionic agents such as Omnipaque (GE Healthcare, Piscataway, New Jersey) are used. Many of us have used these agents for sialography in the past, but this salivary gland investigative technique is labor intensive and has largely been replaced by conventional CT with contrast and MRI for salivary gland evaluation.

We are neither trained to perform these interventions, nor do we require any application for evaluation of head and neck problems with which we deal. Cerebral angiography is used to detect aneurysms, clots that have made their way to the brain giving rise to stroke and other vascular problems. The catheter is inserted into the femoral or carotid artery, and the injected contrast medium administered. The procedure takes hours to perform and must be done in a hospital setting by an interventional radiologist. We will never be trained or licensed to do these procedures. We cannot image vessels in the head and neck region with cone beam technology.

Another "head and neck" radiology task we will never perform is the interpretation of neurologic structures in the brain—at least with CBVT. The exposure factors and the image acquisition technique do not allow us

* 16426 E Emerald Drive, Fountain Hills, AZ 85268.
E-mail address: damilesrad@cox.net

0011-8532/08/$ - see front matter © 2008 Elsevier Inc. All rights reserved.
doi:10.1016/j.cden.2008.06.003   *dental.theclinics.com*

to visualize "gray and white" matter of the brain. In fact, we wouldn't want it to. Again, although many oral and maxillofacial radiologists are "familiar" with the features of disorders and disease affecting the brain such as multiple sclerosis and disseminated herpetic lesions, we are neither trained nor licensed to perform interpretation of these neural structures and problems. And, luckily for us, CBVT cannot image these types of problems. The CBVT machines and techniques are suitable for bone and some soft tissue imaging tasks we require but are vastly inferior to conventional CT for most medical problems.

Finally, it is my opinion that dentists and dental specialists will never completely replace some conventional imaging techniques such as intraoral and panoramic with CBVT.

These restrictions aside, CBVT has opened a new door for all of us in the dental profession. We can now perform limited imaging tasks, like our medical radiology colleagues, with software tools that rival theirs for visualization of anatomy and pathology specifically related to our desired applications. Let's now see what the "future" might hold for us with all of the imaging techniques available. What follows is a series of questions we've been asked or ask ourselves, followed by my "predictions" of how and why oral and maxillofacial imaging techniques will evolve.

Predictions for intraoral, panoramic, and "advanced" imaging modalities

Question #1: Will intraoral and panoramic imaging disappear or be replaced by CBVT?

My response is a resounding, "NO!" Certainly the ability to "slice" through a patient's dental anatomy at 0.15 mm thicknesses could uncover a carious lesion, right? The answer is "Yes" and "No." Although we can see cavitations in some volumes more precisely (Fig. 1), in others the scatter artifact, running horizontally through the occlusal region, will obscure many lesions (Fig. 2). Besides, it is currently, and I think for many years to come, unjustified to use CBVT for caries detection [1,2]. Why you might ask?

First, as low as the x-ray doses are for CBVT machines, the x-ray dose is still too high for many dental imaging tasks. Second, the simpler, more conventional techniques to image interproximal cavities still have the highest resolution. In addition, certain panoramic machines can now provide high-resolution interproximal images, collimated to reduce dose and provide periapical information that may reduce the total number of intraoral images we require for treatment planning (Fig. 3). The large bitewing images below also could replace some posterior intraoral images from the cuspid posteriorly. Note how they even give a detailed view of the third molar region. This would leave only a few anterior views in an initial new patient examination. And, those are the images the auxiliary likes to do!

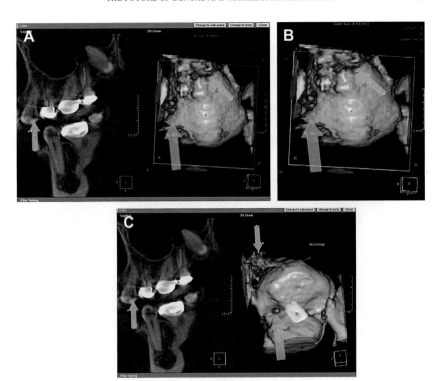

Fig. 1. (*A*) Interproximal carious lesion on the distal of tooth #12. There is some distortion of this area because of scatter artifact from the restorations. The 3D color reconstructions using N-Liten from PlanmecaUSA (Roselle, Illinois). The "Cube Tool" allows better visualization of the lesion in (*B*) (*large blue arrows*). However, the noise artifact created by these restorations is apparent (*small blue arrows*) in 3D views. (*C*) The lesion, although appearing "interproximal" may actually have developed as a "distal pit" lesion as seen in the 3D color view (*large blue arrow*). Noise is again distracting (*small blue arrow*). Case images in Planmeca N-Liten software.

Prediction #1

Although we may use fewer intraoral images, both bitewing and periapical, and even with advances in panoramic techniques and software that can replace some intraoral images, we still will need the higher resolution capability of film or digital intraoral images for high-risk "caries patients" to see the earliest lesions. Cone beam imaging will not replace intraoral or panoramic.

Question #2: Will tomography or panoramic imaging technique be replaced by CBVT?

My response to this question is a hearty "Yes"! Although tomography-was considered "state-of-the-art" for implant planning, even with the best machines and tomographic programs that are available in some panoramic machines, the technique is "labor intensive" once again. Despite the acceptable quality that these images may have, they cannot be made thin enough to precisely locate the alveolar crest in many cases. The technique's

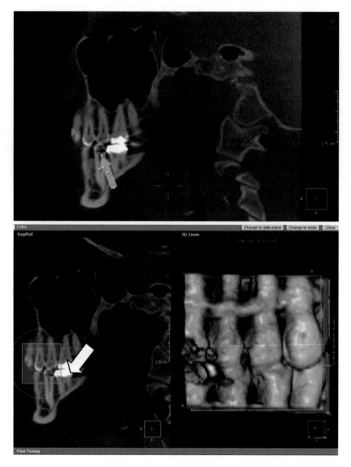

Fig. 2. This volume from an Imaging Sciences i-CAT also shows how even minor scatter artifact from restorations can obscure caries detection. Volume was imaged in OnDemand3D,
(CyberMed International, Seoul, Korea).

magnification factors with either dedicated tomography or panoramic
tomography programs must always be considered. Clinicians still have to
factor in these technique parameters and leave the traditional 2 mm of
"safety margin." With CBVT the measurements are accurate to within
1/10 mm in most software. And, all structures are rendered in a 1:1 ratio
in the image reconstruction software. The margin of error is more precise
with CBVT. You can "recapture" 1 to 1.5 mm of space that might mean
the difference between being able to place a fixture and not being able.

As an aside, many clinicians first encountering CBVT images, and stuck
in their conventional imaging techniques, confuse the term 1:1 ratio with
their perception of "life size!" If the structures are rendered in a precise
1:1 ratio, we can make the image of an implant site into an 8- × 11-inch
glossy print. And if the measured length says 12.2 mm, it IS 12.2 mm to

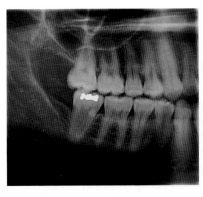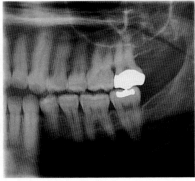

Fig. 3. A bitewing image from a panoramic image capture. Almost all contacts are "open" making caries detection in the bicuspid region possible. This can only be accomplished because of a C-arm on the top of the ProMax (PlanmecaUSA, Roselle, Illinois) panoramic machine, which allows the device to start from a different location and "open" the bicuspid contacts. Currently, in all other panoramic machines these contacts are overlapped and cannot be used for detecting carious lesions interproximally.

within 1/10 of a millimeter! You do not have to use tiny little transparency overlays with implant icon fixtures over a tiny little image of the mandible or maxilla. Those days are gone! That is not the "state-of-the-art" any longer. Images like that in Fig. 4 illustrate this point.

As for panoramic imaging remaining a "standard of care," I can state this. In my opinion it really was never a standard of care. Clinicians, including oral and maxillofacial surgeons, were placing themselves at some risk for using a panoramic image as the sole radiographic means of implant site assessment. Some still do. Now that CBVT has become so widely available, the use of a panoramic image, with the myriad of positioning errors made and the lack of the cross-sectional information cannot be justified. Anyone who persists using this image as their only image for implant site

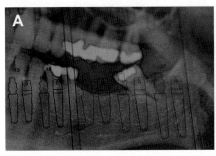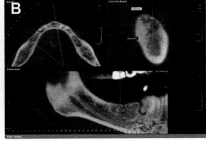

Fig. 4. (A) A panoramic image with a "transparency overlay" of generic implant icons. (Courtesy of Ronald Shelley, DMD, Glendale, AZ). (B) A typical cross-sectional display with nerve marked in red and precise measurements labeled on the proposed implant site for tooth #30 (implant image #83). If needed, an icon can be overlayed to better visualize the proposed site.

evaluation will have a serious liability issue in my opinion. Fig. 5A–D show the improved information available with CBVT technique software.

> *Prediction #2*
>   *CBVT will replace conventional tomography as the "standard of care," and should now be used in place of panoramic imaging to assess any implant site.*

Question #3: Will CBVT replace conventional CT as the "state-of-the-art" or the "standard of care" for presurgical implant site evaluation?

Yes. Period! With the substantially reduced patient x-ray dose [3], the "implant-specific" software, the smaller voxel size, the wider "availability" and the reduced cost, CBVT will become the standard of care within the foreseeable future. This is obvious from the images seen above.

> *Prediction #3*
>   *CBVT will replace conventional CT as the standard of care for implant assessment.*

Question #4: Will the "cephalometric" image reconstructed from a CBVT data volume replace the conventional cephalometric image for cephalometric analysis?

My answer today is "not yet." Since the 1940s when the cephalometric techniques were introduced, orthodontists have developed many ways of

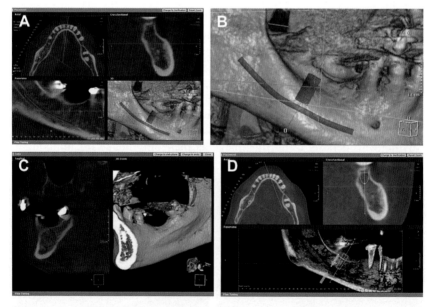

Fig. 5. (*A*) Typical implant planning image set shows a "generic" implant fixture orientation in relation to the inferior alveolar nerve. (*B*) A close-up image of the case above isolating the 3D color volume and proposed implant placement visualization. (*C*) A 3D colorized view to show the submandibular fossa in relation to the implant site. (*D*) A colorized "slab" rendering allows the clinician to actually see the canal and the desired position of the intended implant fixture. Precise measurements can now be made.

performing an "analysis" of the conventional cephalometric image to predict final tooth position and have been using these "analyses" for more than 60 years. Today, in the dental profession, just because a technology is available in the marketplace does not mean it can immediately replace the current "standard." This was obvious from the discussion above. However, in orthodontics, this is especially true. As dentistry's first specialty, orthodontics has had a long history of examining and developing the "clinical science" behind their orthodontic analyses. In my opinion, here's what will and should happen before CBVT completely replaces conventional cephalometric techniques.

With the push in dentistry for evidence-based dentistry, multipatient, multitrial research will need to be completed. Possibly 50 patients at each of 10 dental schools or other sites will need to have their traditional cephalometric analyses performed on conventional "cephs" compared with a matching number of patients at each site whose cephalometric image(s) are reconstructed by CBVT software. Then these patients will need to be followed up for 5 years to see if the CBVT technique is more precise than the conventional technique for predicting final tooth position. My gut feeling is that CBVT will outperform conventional cephalometric measurement. Why? The main reason is the fact that, the image data, as stated earlier, is reconstructed at a precise 1:1 ratio. As a result, the magnification artifact(s) inherent in conventional cephalometric x-ray techniques are eliminated. Thus, the localization of the typical landmarks used in the analyses will be more precise, reduced operator error. So, the adoption of CBVT for orthodontic cephalometric analyses is inevitable. Software manufacturers are just now beginning to create the software to perform these analyses. I do not believe orthodontists are ready to "give up" their traditional analyses just yet.

Prediction #4

CBVT will replace conventional cephalometric x-ray technique as the standard of care within 7 to 10 years after the "science" has been completed.

Question #5: Will CBVT imaging replace panoramic imaging for third molar extraction?

In my opinion, my answer would be "not completely." Not every impacted third molar is located close to anatomic entities that could cause problems like the inferior alveolar nerve (IAN) or the maxillary antra. Some are; some are not (Fig. 6). If an oral and maxillofacial surgeon can obtain the initial information on a panoramic image, film, or digital image, and if the teeth to be removed are in locations that do not approximate the sinuses or IANs, then the clinical treatment decision s simple, the panoramic image provides the necessary data by itself, and CBVT may not be required. They may not even require a "large-volume" machine. If the machine is capable of capturing both the panoramic image alone (low dose to patient) and CBVT data (higher dose to patient), then the decision making

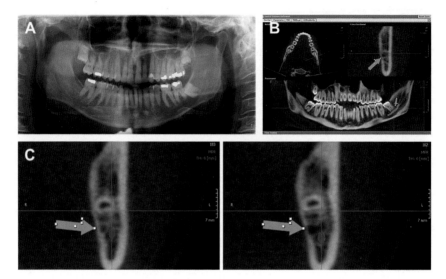

Fig. 6. (*A*) This excellent digital panoramic reveals 3 impacted molars. If only the upper molars were impacted, a CBVT volume may not be necessary. However, the lower left third molar does appear to be in close proximity to the IAN, so a CBVT should be ordered. Some machines like the ProMax3D can do both using CBVT volume only when needed. (*B*) This "pseudopanoramic" from an i-CAT volume has the nerve colorized and shows the developing apex of tooth #17 touching the IAN. (*C*) These cross-sectional images of tooth #17 show the proximity of the IAN to additional root areas of the tooth touching the IAN.

is improved as well as the productivity. In an oral and maxillofacial surgeon's office, time is money, and surgical removal of third molars is the primary procedure. Many oral and maxillofacial surgeons do not want to wait for image reconstruction from CBVT machines (as quick as they may have become) to see a panoramic view in a simple case.

Prediction #5
CBVT will replace conventional panoramic images as the standard of care only for difficult third molar extraction cases.

Future considerations for cone beam volumetric tomography imaging

This is perhaps the most difficult area to make any predictions about because of the ingenuity and creativity of the dental software companies. New, innovative software technology is introduced constantly to our profession. Dentists are more and more computer literate and find processes and tasks in their own offices they wish to simplify or streamline.

Here are the primary areas for growth and thus predictions for dental imaging in the future. Most future uses, obviously, are related to CBVT.

- Software improvement
- Image-to-device processes

- Picture archiving and communication systems (PACS)/ radiographic information systems (RIS)

Software improvement(s)

Software from the machine manufacturers is already good. They could not have introduced their hardware without accompanying software and be successful. However, some of the manufacturers have proprietary software. Examples are Imaging Sciences International (i-CAT, Hatfield, Pennsylvania) and AFP Imaging (NewTom 3G and VG, Elmsford, New York). Although both these machines—as all other CBCT machines—can export their volume data to third party software, DICOM (digital imaging and communication in medicine) data cannot be imported into the manufacturer's software for use with their templates and reporting tools. Although not a serious drawback, it is a point to consider when purchasing or using these machines. Third-party software is the biggest area of "growth" and is discussed below.

The most robust type of three-dimensional (3D) color software would include several parameters to assign to the voxel information. Every manufacturer and third-party software can handle the two-dimensional (2D) grayscale assignment to the voxel. Some even have algorithms to approximate Houndsfield units. Some third-party software can also perform surface rendering of the voxel units assigning a color to the voxel. You have seen many examples of gold, green, and even purple mandibles in implant planning software programs. A few vendors, for example Planmeca (Romexis, Helsinki, Finland) and Imaging Sciences (3DVR, Hatfield, Pennsylvania) and can assign a transparency value to each voxel to make a seemingly "transparent" image. A third-party company, Anatomage (San Jose, California) has this type of software and has created products for cephalometric landmark AnatoCeph tracing and implant planning (In Vivo Dental software, Anatomage, Inc., San Jose, California). Fig. 7 shows some of these products.

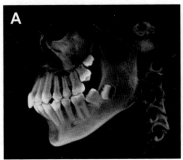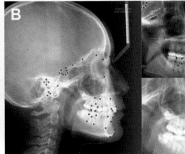

Fig. 7. (*A*) Typical 3D color reconstruction software with color and transparency shows course of IAN canal through the mandible. (*B*) Cephalometric tracing. (*Courtesy of* Anatomage, San Jose, CA. Available at: http://www.anatomage.com. Accessed June 27, 2008; with permission.)

The highest level of software treatment is able to assign color, transparency, and opacity values to the CBVT voxel information. To date, only OnDemand3D (CyberMed International, Seoul, Korea) can perform these tasks (Fig. 8).

Table 1 shows some of these third-party companies' products and capability.

Useful software improvements

1. All software will be able to assign all 3 attributes—color, transparency, and opacity
2. Improved "scatter rejection" algorithms
3. All software completely DICOM compliant
4. Software in four dimensions to create the "Virtual Articulator"
5. Online, Internet "portal" software to speed surgical guide construction and delivery as well as interpretive reports and analytic images (eg, measured implant sites)
6. PACS/RIS systems for dentistry (see discussion below)

Picture archiving and communication systems/radiographic information system radiographic information delivery

PACS have been developed and used in medicine for many years. The ability to store, retrieve, and share image information between medical specialists, including radiologists payers, administrators, and others, has

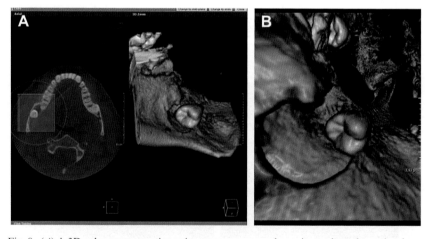

Fig. 8. (A) A 3D color reconstruction using transparency and opacity to show the occlusal surface of the third molar impacted in the bone! (Image created with OnDemand3D "Cube" tool, CyberMed, Seoul, Korea). (B) Same tooth as shown above but imaged with CyberMed's "endoscopy" tool. Note the cuspal and developmental groove anatomy.

Table 1
Oral and maxillofacial products and manufacturers

Manufacturer	Product name	Web site URL	Primary software task(s)
3dMD	3dMDFace 3DMD Cranial	http://www.3dmd.com/home.asp	Orthodontics
Anatomage	In Vivo Dental AnatoCeph	http://www.anatomage.com/home.htm	Implant, ortho
CyberMed	OnDemand3D Vworks Vceph	http://www.cybermed.co.kr/eindex.php	Multiple
Dolphin	Dolphin 3D (OEM from Anatomage)	http://www.dolphinimaging.com/ new_site/home.html	Orthodontics
NobelBioCare	NobelGuide	http://www.nobelbiocare.com/global/en/	Implant
Materialise Dental	SimPlant	http://www.materialise.com/materialise/ view/en/84113-Dental+homepage.html	Implant

grown an entire industry for these tasks. Until now, dentistry had only a couple of such products, and they were not widely used. Indeed, in the best of worlds, medical and dental records could be shared and distributed using PACS systems.

RIS is really just the information highway to deliver the radiologist's report to the referring hospital, clinician, or colleague. The two systems or products really go hand in hand.

Now there is a PACS/RIS product specifically for dentistry. CyberMed's OnDemand PACS/RIS was designed to handle the necessary data volumes, deliver reports, and analyses and archive client data off-site, one of the many, necessary Health Insurance Portability and Accountability Act (HIPAA) regulations. To date, it is the only HIPAA-compliant product I know of to use with our CBVT volumes. Remember that each patient case is 60 to 250 MB, depending on machine manufacturer. These large files must be moved quickly, safely, and efficiently without corruption. Dentistry has truly "made it to the big time" with this capability.

The PACS/RIS also does a lot more. Think of it as a "Practice Management System" for the office or laboratory. All dentists using cone beam, cone beam imaging laboratories, and single cone beam will use a PACS/RIS within 5 years.

Image-to-device processes

Perhaps the most exciting area of dental and maxillofacial imaging will come in the area of device manufacture from 3D data using an "Online Distributive Network." Dentists want to be able to request or order radiographic stents, surgical guides, study and orthodontic models, and other devices directly from their office computers.

Companies currently are raising venture capital to deliver these appliances and devices electronically. The Cone Beam image data makes this possible. Already we can see the patient's 3D color dentition. Many clinicians are sending their patient's data for surgical guide construction through companies like NobelBiocare. Larger surgical guides, requiring temporary horizontal "anchorage" to place multiple fixtures for overdentures can be received by mail or courier delivery. But, many more services, including faster, simpler delivery for single implant cases, will soon be offered through "Internet Portals" or distributive networks because of CBVT imaging. There are many more simple cases than complex cases.

Summary

In summary, CBVT, as good as it is and will be, is a complementary technique to other more conventional imaging technologies. It offers our profession a substantial improvement for some but not all of our imaging tasks or need. For some procedures, it will become the standard of care.

Improvements in software removal of scatter artifacts; reduced x-ray dose; and delivery of interpretive reports, analyses, appliances, and images will continue, and use of CBVT will increase. Distributive networks will be introduced to simplify all of these tasks. Virtual articulators, computer assisted design and computer assisted manufacturing devices will improve, and online delivery of some of these services will increase concomitantly. In all, dentistry will improve and, along with it, patient care.

References

[1] Miles DA, Danforth RA. A clinician's guide to understanding cone beam volumetric imaging. Academy of Dental Therapeutics and Stomatology. Available at: www.ineedce.com.
[2] Haiter-Neto F, Wenzel A, Gotfredsen E. Diagnostic accuracy of cone beam computed tomography scans compared with intraoral imaging modalities for detection of caries. Dentomaxillofac Radiol 2008;37:18–22.
[3] Suomalainen A, Vehmas T, Kortesniemi M, et al. Accuracy of linear measurements using dental cone beam and conventional multislice computed tomography. Dentomaxillofac Radiol 2008;37:10–7.

ELSEVIER
SAUNDERS

Dent Clin N Am 52 (2008) 929–933

THE DENTAL
CLINICS
OF NORTH AMERICA

Index

Note: Page numbers of article titles are in **boldface** type.

doi:10.1016/S0011-8532(08)00063-3
dental.theclinics.com

Tomography, conventional, of
    temporomandibular joint, 878
    or panoramic imaging, cone beam
        volumetric tomography and,
        919–922
    plain film, compared with cone-beam
        CT imaging, 848–849

Tuned aperture CT, 826

U

Ultrasonography, of temporomandibular
    joint, 880

V

Vertebra, C3, and hyoid, cone-beam CT
    imaging at level of, 736–737, 739, 740

Virtual models, cone-beam CT imaging and,
    801–804, 818–819

Moving?

Make sure your subscription moves with you!

To notify us of your new address, find your **Clinics Account Number** (located on your mailing label above your name), and contact customer service at:

E-mail: elspcs@elsevier.com

800-654-2452 (subscribers in the U.S. & Canada)
1-407-563-6020 (subscribers outside of the U.S. & Canada)

Fax number: 407-363-9661

Elsevier Periodicals Customer Service
6277 Sea Harbor Drive
Orlando, FL 32887-4800

*To ensure uninterrupted delivery of your subscription, please notify us at least 4 weeks in advance of move.

United States Postal Service

Statement of Ownership, Management, and Circulation
(All Periodicals Publications Except Requestor Publications)

1. Publication Title	2. Publication Number		3. Filing Date
Dental Clinics of North America	5 6 6 - 4 8 0		9/15/08

4. Issue Frequency	5. Number of Issues Published Annually	6. Annual Subscription Price
Jan, Apr, Jul, Oct	4	$188.00

7. Complete Mailing Address of Known Office of Publication *(Not printer) (Street, city, county, state, and ZIP+4)*

Elsevier Inc.
360 Park Avenue South
New York, NY 10010-1710

Contact Person
Stephen Bushing
Telephone (include area code)
215-239-3688

8. Complete Mailing Address of Headquarters or General Business Office of Publisher *(Not printer)*

Elsevier Inc., 360 Park Avenue South, New York, NY 10010-1710

9. Full Names and Complete Mailing Addresses of Publisher, Editor, and Managing Editor *(Do not leave blank)*

Publisher *(Name and complete mailing address)*

John Schrefer, Elsevier, Inc., 1600 John F. Kennedy Blvd. Suite 1800, Philadelphia, PA 19103-2899

Editor *(Name and complete mailing address)*

John Vassallo, Elsevier, Inc., 1600 John F. Kennedy Blvd. Suite 1800, Philadelphia, PA 19103-2899

Managing Editor *(Name and complete mailing address)*

Catherine Bewick, Elsevier, Inc., 1600 John F. Kennedy Blvd. Suite 1800, Philadelphia, PA 19103-2899

10. Owner *(Do not leave blank. If the publication is owned by a corporation, give the name and address of the corporation immediately followed by the names and addresses of all stockholders owning or holding 1 percent or more of the total amount of stock. If not owned by a corporation, give the names and addresses of the individual owners. If owned by a partnership or other unincorporated firm, give its name and address as well as those of each individual owner. If the publication is published by a nonprofit organization, give its name and address.)*

Full Name	Complete Mailing Address
Wholly owned subsidiary of	4520 East-West Highway
Reed/Elsevier, US holdings	Bethesda, MD 20814

11. Known Bondholders, Mortgages, and Other Security Holders Owning or Holding 1 Percent or More of Total Amount of Bonds, Mortgages, or Other Securities. If none, check box ☐ None

Full Name	Complete Mailing Address
N/A	

12. Tax Status *(For completion by nonprofit organizations authorized to mail at nonprofit rates) (Check one)*
The purpose, function, and nonprofit status of this organization and the exempt status for federal income tax purposes:
☐ Has Not Changed During Preceding 12 Months
☐ Has Changed During Preceding 12 Months *(Publisher must submit explanation of change with this statement)*

PS Form 3526, September 2006 (Page 1 of 3 (Instructions Page 3)) PSN 7530-01-000-9931 **PRIVACY NOTICE:** See our Privacy policy in www.usps.com

13. Publication Title	14. Issue Date for Circulation Data Below
Dental Clinics of North America	July 2008

15. Extent and Nature of Circulation		Average No. Copies Each Issue During Preceding 12 Months	No. Copies of Single Issue Published Nearest to Filing Date
a. Total Number of Copies *(Net press run)*		2150	2100
b. Paid Circulation (By Mail and Outside the Mail)	(1) Mailed Outside-County Paid Subscriptions Stated on PS Form 3541. *(Include paid distribution above nominal rate, advertiser's proof copies, and exchange copies)*	999	945
	(2) Mailed In-County Paid Subscriptions Stated on PS Form 3541 *(Include paid distribution above nominal rate, advertiser's proof copies, and exchange copies)*		
	(3) Paid Distribution Outside the Mails Including Sales Through Dealers and Carriers, Street Vendors, Counter Sales, and Other Paid Distribution Outside USPS®	428	447
	(4) Paid Distribution by Other Classes Mailed Through the USPS (e.g. First-Class Mail®)		
c. Total Paid Distribution *(Sum of 15b (1), (2), (3), and (4))*	▶	1427	1392
d. Free or Nominal Rate Distribution (By Mail and Outside the Mail)	(1) Free or Nominal Rate Outside-County Copies Included on PS Form 3541	64	98
	(2) Free or Nominal Rate In-County Copies Included on PS Form 3541		
	(3) Free or Nominal Rate Copies Mailed at Other Classes Mailed Through the USPS (e.g. First-Class Mail)		
	(4) Free or Nominal Rate Distribution Outside the Mail (Carriers or other means)		
e. Total Free or Nominal Rate Distribution (Sum of 15d (1), (2), (3) and (4))	▶	64	98
f. Total Distribution (Sum of 15c and 15e)	▶	1491	1490
g. Copies not Distributed *(See instructions to publishers #4 (page #3))*	▶	659	610
h. Total (Sum of 15f and g)	▶	2150	2100
i. Percent Paid (15c divided by 15f times 100)		95.71%	93.42%

16. Publication of Statement of Ownership
☐ If the publication is a general publication, publication of this statement is required. Will be printed in the **October 2008** issue of this publication. ☐ Publication not required.

17. Signature and Title of Editor, Publisher, Business Manager, or Owner
[signature]
John Vassallo – Executive Director of Subscription Services

Date
September 15, 2008

I certify that all information furnished on this form is true and complete. I understand that anyone who furnishes false or misleading information on this form or who omits material or information requested on the form may be subject to criminal sanctions (including fines and imprisonment) and/or civil sanctions (including civil penalties).

PS Form 3526, September 2006 (Page 2 of 3)